FIRESIDE

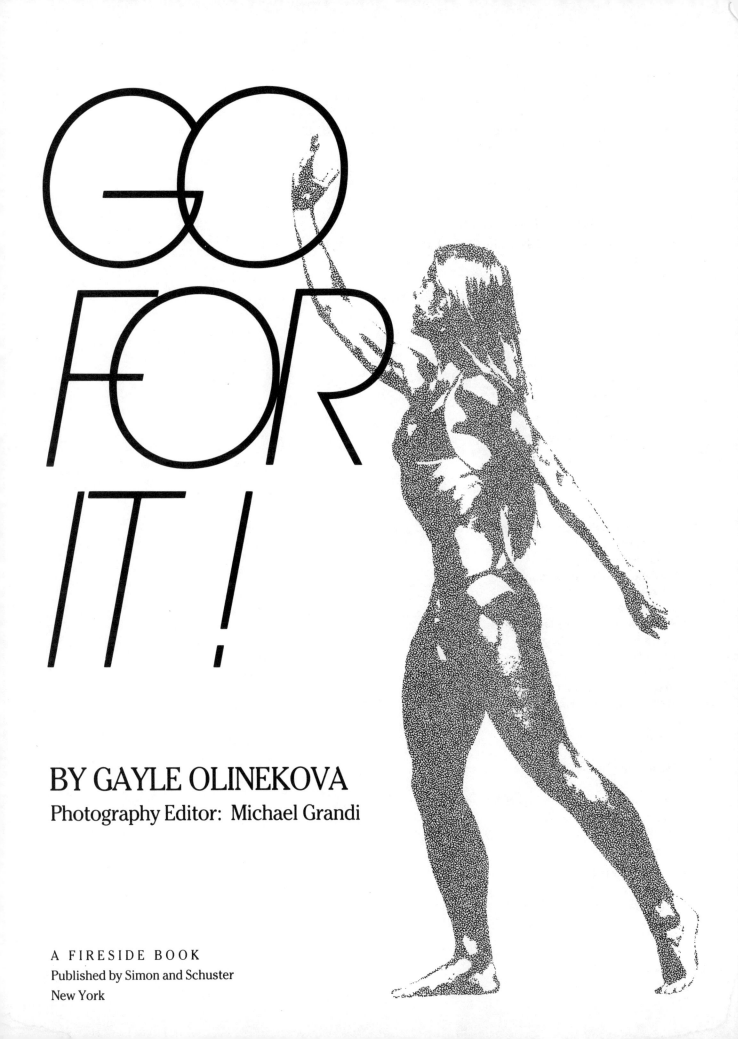

GO FOR IT!

BY GAYLE OLINEKOVA
Photography Editor: Michael Grandi

A FIRESIDE BOOK
Published by Simon and Schuster
New York

Photo credits

Richard Mackson: front cover, x, 38, 86, 91, 104, 144, 145, 146, 147, 148 top, 151

Michael Grandi: iii, 4 bottom, 18 bottom, 22, 80 left, 85, 121 left, 133, 153, 157, 164

Carol Guzy: vii, 3

Women's Track World: 2

Lady Athlete: 4 top, 10, 166

Drew Levitan: 5 bottom, 121 side shot, 124 top, 143

Art Seitz: 6 bottom, 7, 11, 13, 14, 15, 16, 17, 21, 24, 78, 80 top, 82, 94, 98, 102, 103, 111, 114, 131, 140

John Balik: 8, 120, 123, 128, 130

Bill Heimanson: 9, 23, 132, 134, 135, 138, 148 bottom, 149 top

Janeart: 12, 20

Robert Riger: 18 top, 127

Rick Semple: 19, 122, 136, 137, 139, 149 bottom

Don Lauritzen: 27–37, 39–77, 79, 83, 84, 117, 126 top, 129, 152

Charles Suter: viii

Richard Slotkin: 126 bottom

Line drawings by Charles Suter

A Fireside Book
Published by Simon and Schuster
A Division of Gulf & Western Corporation
Simon & Schuster Building
Rockefeller Center
1230 Avenue of the Americas
New York, New York 10020
FIRESIDE and colophon are registered trademarks of Simon & Schuster

Designed by H. Roberts Design

Manufactured in the United States of America
10 9 8 7 6 5 4 3 2 1
Library of Congress Cataloging in Publication Data

Olinekova, Gayle,
  Go for it!

  "A Fireside book."
  Bibliography: p.
  1. Physical fitness. 2. Exercise. 3. Nutrition.
I. Title.
GV481.035   1982   613.7   82-16775

ISBN: 0-671-45692-X

ACKNOWLEDGMENTS

Life as an amateur athlete does mean being alone on the roads, but through all the long miles and all the years of training, there are those whose unfailing generosity, loving kindness and inspirational support must be acknowledged.

Ted and Shayla Abood, Lyle Alzado, Dr. Yolande Balestra, George Butler, Kathy and Jan Cook, Louis and Vina D'Agostino, Terri Dalton, Jane Davies, Al DiNoble, Dr. George and Dottie Dorion, Hully Fetico, Manny Gutierrez, Ray Hatch, Kiou Jalayer, Allan Kalmus, Jack Kavanagh, Jim Kupcho, Dan Levin, Franziska Naegli, Mike McConvey, Harvey Mednick, Paul Owens, Dr. Joseph Polacco, Peter Ratazzi, Vreni Roth, Alexis Schade, Leonard Sillman, Al Thomas, Tony Urbaitis, David Zelon, and of course, my family.

My Pit Crew. CAPTAIN—Dr. JACK KAHN, Chiropractor, Dr. Kenneth Rehm, Podiatrist, Dr. Michael Grandi, Naturopath, Bill Speizman, Physical Therapy, Johanna Klamer.

Consultants. Dan Altchuler, DPM, Adrian Grice, DC, Rob Krakovitz, MD, John Pagliano, DPM.

Photographers. Exercise photographs by Don Lauritzen, John Balik, Michael Grandi, Bill Heimanson, Drew Levitan, Art Seitz, Rick Semple, Richard Mackson.

Cover Photography. Richard Mackson, *Sports Illustrated.*

Artist. Charles Suter.

A special thanks to the following gyms: Bath Beach Gym, Coral Springs Health Spa, Gold's Gym, Gold Coast Gym, and World Gym.

Typing. Edith Butler.

Chart on page 88 from *The Bermuda Inn.*

There are others, too numerous to mention, who have cheered me and cheered for me. There are some whose lives are singularly an example of courage in the face of challenge—not the publicized public figures of our times, but the "little people" who carry on regardless—heroes in their own right. And finally, there are some whose death has inspired me to reach for the top, so that their sacrifices would not be in vain.

To all of you, my deepest thanks.

The following books were helpful as references in researching the book.

Materia Medica by William Boericke, M.D.

Back to Eden by Jethro Kloss

Survival Into the Twenty-first Century by Viktoras Kulvinskas

DEDICATION

To my darling Michael—without whom this book
would still be just another Aries dream

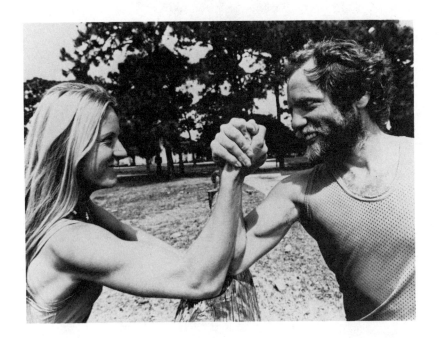

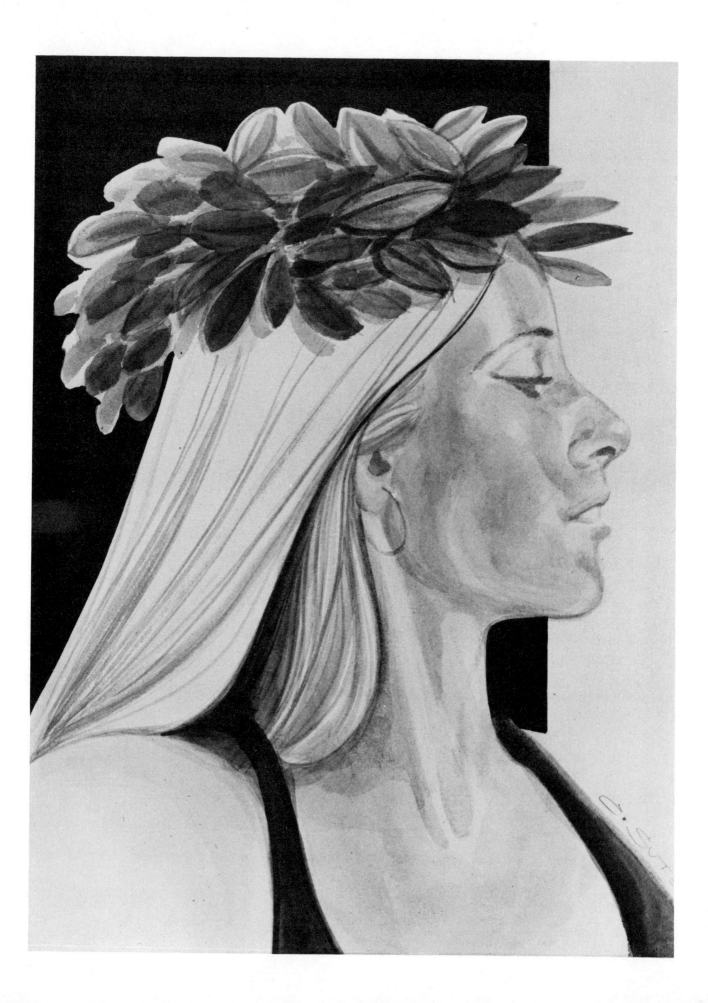

CONTENTS

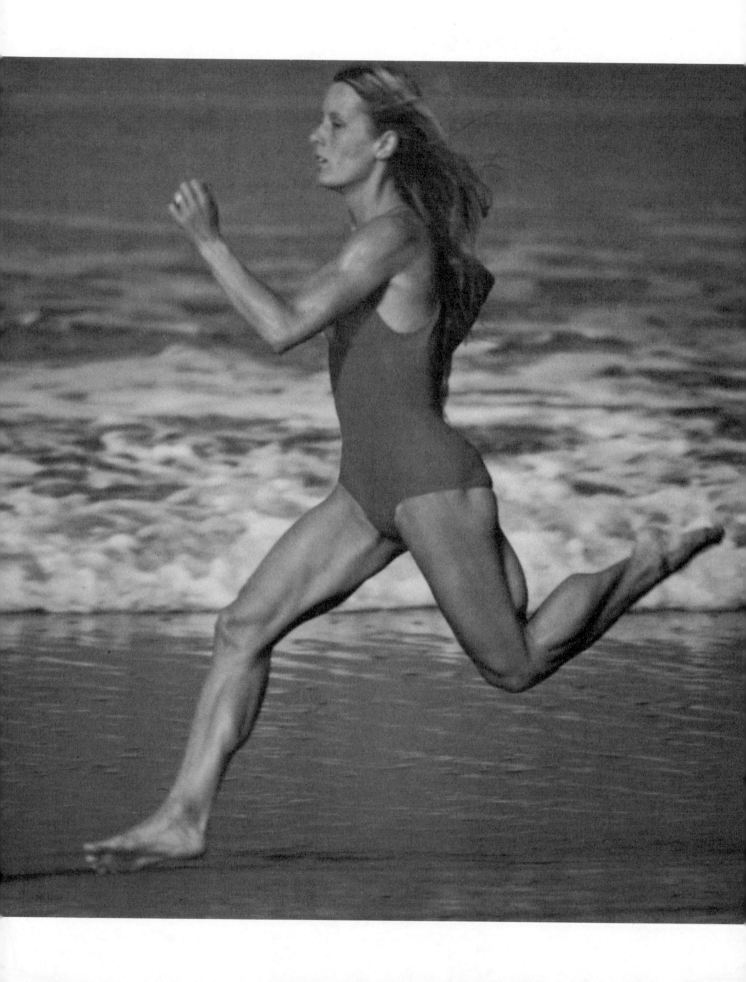

GO FOR IT!
AN INTRODUCTION

Whatever you can do, or dream you can, begin it.
Boldness has genius, power and magic in it.

Goethe

On Christmas Eve, 1968, I promised myself that I would go for it. I loved to run and decided to put all my energies into that. I didn't even own a pair of running shoes.

Eight months later, at the age of sixteen, I was National Champion in the quarter mile and on my way to Tokyo to compete in the first Pan Pacific Games. I remember climbing onto the victory podium to get my bronze metal and thinking, "Now I really have to learn how to train."

That took longer than I ever expected. Injury and mononucleosis from overtraining with my first two coaches made me realize that my overwhelming desire and effort were not enough. I needed to learn the why and how of getting stronger and winning.

After touring Europe as an 800-meter runner in 1972, I narrowly missed the 1972 Olympic team by a few tenths of a second. I was nominated outstanding female junior athlete of the year, but was disappointed. Something different was needed.

I put sprinting on hold and used a scholarship to enroll in college, having decided that the fine arts program had a lot to offer—modern dance. I had never danced anything in my life except a polka at my grandparents' fiftieth wedding anniversary, but the audition for this program was so crowded (476 hopefuls for 30 spots) I felt that there was nothing to lose. I was no match for all those nascent prima ballerinas, but I made it. The dance master said that I was different and new, with a style all my own.

Modern dance was like discovering sex for the first time. I never knew that moving your body could feel so beautiful and sensual. As a newcomer, the other dancers resented me at first, but then choreographed dramatic pieces for me that highlighted my strength and speed—high leaps, turns and bounding. It was hard work but extremely gratifying.

In February 1973 I was selected for the Canada vs. U.S.S.R. track meet. I began to run again in earnest. The front page photo of the *Montreal Star* for March 25 showed me outleaning Gerisamova of the Soviet Union—an Olympic finalist.

Dance had taught me that strength plus flexibility equals speed. To complement my strength, I had taken up speed skating, which made me conscious of the low back and gluteus muscles as a source of power to the body.

Still, I needed to learn more. Late in 1973, frustrated in my efforts to learn new things, I made plans to leave Canada. I had $150 to my

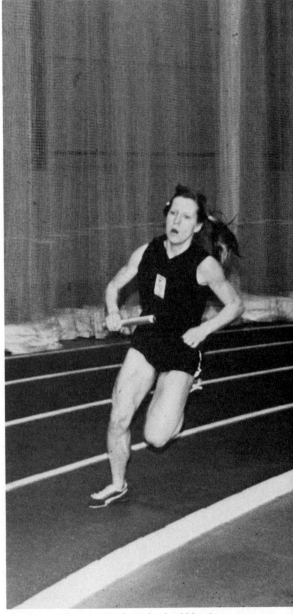

Anchoring the winning leg of a 4 x 100 relay indoors. Quebec City, 1970

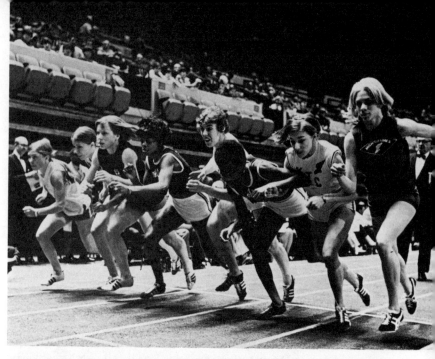

Madison Square Garden's 1970 Olympic Invitational. At the start of the 880 yards, I'm third from the left.

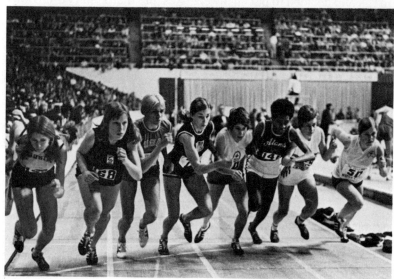

Toronto Star Games, 1969. One of the fastest indoor half-miles ever assembled, including Cheryl Toussant, third from the right, and Francie Kraker-Johnson, third from the left. I'm second from the left.

name and bought a one-way ticket to Amsterdam for $100. Surely in Europe I would find out what I needed to know. Maybe a sport hypnotist or a famous doctor. I had yet to explore the mental aspects of sport. I felt I needed life experience. I got both in an almost two-year odyssey that saw me push myself mentally and physically beyond the periphery of anything I had known to that time.

I traveled to the sport science centers in Switzerland, Germany, Italy and France, waiting sometimes for hours before the famous scientists would deign to answer even one question. I studied German in order to understand East German translations of Soviet sports documents.

In the summer of 1974 I was hired as a lumberjack in the forests of Switzerland—the only woman among hundreds of men. On August 18, after ten hours of labor, I traveled to Zurich and won the 800 meters in the most prestigious track meet in Europe—the Weltklasse Invitational.

I viewed the pampered European athletes with respect for their achievements, but also felt something bordering on disdain. They had the best of everything—coaches, trainers, doctors, facilities. Their only job was to compete and succeed in sports, and I was glad to beat

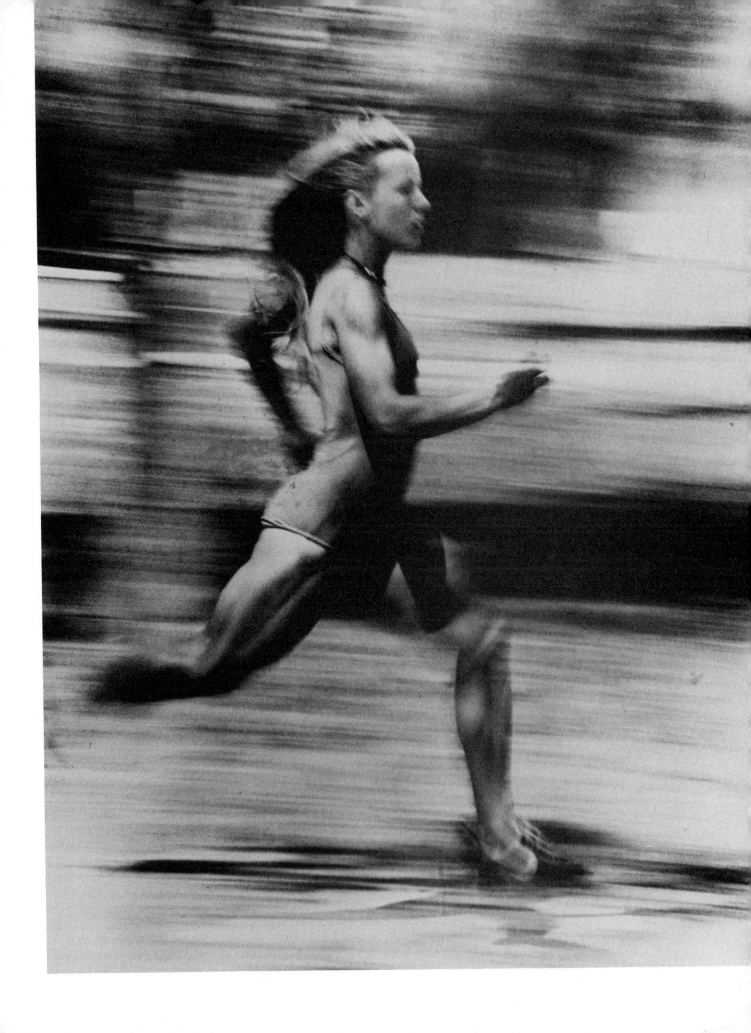

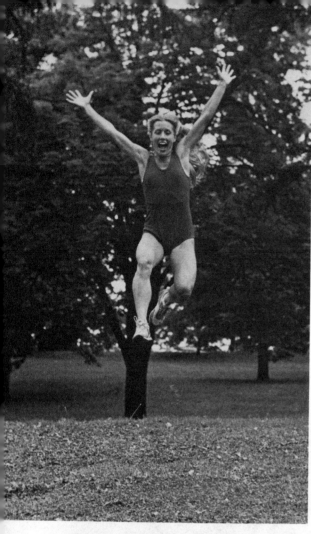

them at their own game. In one way I envied them the assurance that their talent would always be consummated in the most successful way known. Their every whim was catered to, psychologists prepared their minds for the race, coaches hovered over them like surrogate mothers. But did they know why they won, or understand how?

Just two years before, to win would have been enough for me, but now I had to know the why of it and to be able to duplicate the effort again and again—and to do it by myself. I nearly killed myself trying.

I felt invincible, and hitchhiked toward Africa with the intention of going to Kenya to train at high altitude the way the great Kenyan Olympic champions had. I was too inexperienced to know that wins such as those at the Weltklasse—miracle wins—can occasionally be pulled out of your entrails, but you can't expect your body to perform at that high level without some backup: regular food and sleep for instance.

I picked grapes near Geneva to finance the trip—long grueling hours in the cold rain—going for runs after eleven-hour days in the fields. Here I learned where the term "back-breaking" was invented. However, my upper body and low back became stronger with the work, and I was running faster at night even though exhausted. Now I understood why the Europeans put so much emphasis on gymnastics and upper body work in their training—it benefits speed.

A bout of cholera in Marseilles and civil war in Africa delayed my plans. Occasionally, as my strength returned, I ran barefoot in Spain and Morocco until one day I decided to return to North America to recover and chase my dream of making the 1976 Olympic Team.

I concentrated on the 1500 meters—figuring that adding stamina to my speed would be a winning combination. My heart sank when it grew increasingly more difficult to run faster. I tried harder and occasionally pulled out a good performance: third at the Martin Luther King Freedom Games, qualifying times for the Olympic Trials and a big win at the Belgian National Championships.

Two years later I found out that the cholera I had had in Europe had left lingering effects. In the meantime, I realized that I knew next to nothing about food and nutrition—how to heal the body as well as fuel it, and how to strengthen and protect it.

In the fall of 1976, I met Dr. Michael Grandi, a nutritionist and doctor of naturopathy—and a competitive athlete. He was the mentor I had been searching for. I'd never had a cavity in my life, and had never eaten junk food, but he taught me how to combine proper food, a constructive eating schedule with fasting, and appropriate vitamins —the answers for maximum good health.

Eating correctly, I saw the results in a short time: I had more energy, I healed quickly, and from the day I met Michael I never got sick although I had been plagued with bronchitis and colds since childhood.

And then the test. A severe car smashup had doctors telling me I'd never walk again. They wanted to operate on a mangled knee and assorted chips and fractures. I refused. I had just spent seven years learning about my body. I didn't trust it with someone wielding a scalpel.

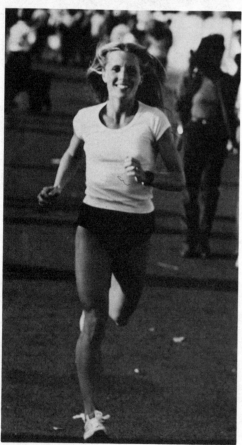

I left Canada for a warmer climate, and sixteen weeks after the accident I began jogging. The scar tissue seemed to just fade away with the sun and good eating—a diet of 95 percent raw foods.

Less than twenty weeks after the accident I ran in the Greater Miami Marathon, planning only to pace Michael for seven miles, but

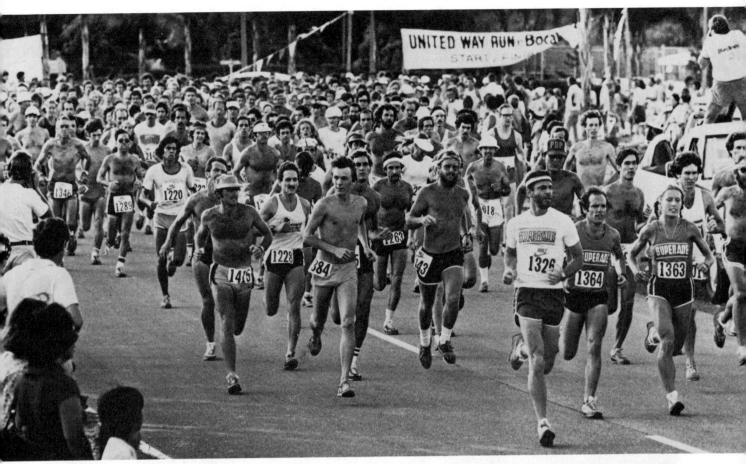

feeling terrific and finishing the whole 26.2 miles—and winning. It seemed too incredible to believe. To prove it wasn't a fluke, I ran another marathon four weeks later and won it (the Fort Myers Marathon), deciding to run the Boston Marathon one month later. I only hoped to finish—and stood at the back of the pack of some 5000 runners. It took me almost five minutes to pass the famous Boston starting line because of the huge crowd, and a ten-minute first mile before I really began to run at a decent pace.

I finished in 2 hours, 56 minutes—fourth place and a Canadian national record. I was only seconds behind the third-place woman and had no idea. Mickey Gorman won in 2:48. The lesson here was: Don't underestimate yourself by standing at the back of the pack. In my "marathon career" my improvement had been more than thirty-five minutes in less than twelve weeks.

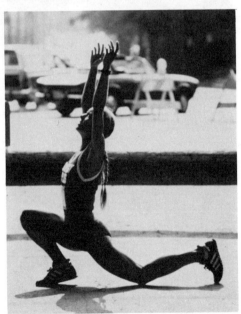

I stayed at near that time for two years, experimenting in what seemed like a vacuum while studying for a degree in nutrition. The running magazines offered no help at all. I was lifting weights and all the experts said don't lift weights. I felt the need to do sprintwork, which the experts also wrote against.

After winning the Orange Bowl Marathon in 1979 (2:55), I decided a change was in order. I gave myself four weeks of fast, hard, brutal workouts, lifted weights, did thousands of sit-ups. We did a time trial on the Orange Bowl course two weeks after the race—2:45. The next week we did it again—this time 2:44.

I felt confident that I would surpass 2:40 in a competitive situation, and at the end of the fourth week I entered the Mardi Gras Marathon and won—2:38:12. This made me the seventh fastest in the world and

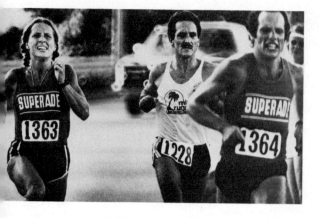

was no surprise to me, but it was a shock to the running world that I could improve fifteen minutes in the marathon in four weeks.

Financial problems and a hot tropical summer weakened my preparations for the World Championships in Germany—sixth place in 2:44. I was disgusted. Now to really follow my instincts. Michael had a Golden Gloves boxing career behind him. I had dance, speedskating, cycling and cross-country skiing disciplines to draw from. Together we formulated a bizarre and unique training program in which I trained more like a prizefighter than a marathon runner.

Because the workouts concentrated on strength, my body changed and I added sleek muscle and sinew to my upper body. I stretched and sweated through old modern dance routines using ankle weights in the afternoon, and ran waist deep in the ocean at night. The mornings I reserved for jumping rope and lifting weights— sometimes hundreds of repetitions for biceps and triceps alone. I disregarded all the "expert" advice I had been given by marathon coaches and athletes. I had done their programs and failed. My body was different and therefore needed completely different workouts.

Ten weeks after the World Championships I ran the Fiesta Bowl Marathon and won in 2:36:12. I was now fifth in the world with a time that would have won the Germany race. I was ranked third in the world for 1979, but felt robbed because a strong headwind cut into my time.

Eight weeks later, I planned another race—the Mardi Gras Marathon again. I followed the same regime but added shorter races. In January 1980, I ran a 20 km race in Florida in 1 hour, 9 minutes—the second fastest time in the world ever—and won the whole race, beating all the women *and* all the men. On February 18 I finished the Mardi

Rough-water rowing with world record holder Erik Jersted. The Atlantic Ocean

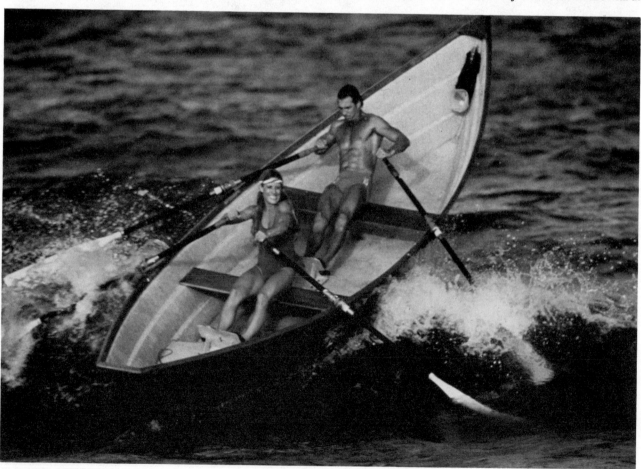

Gras Marathon in 2:35:09 to become the third fastest woman in the history of the marathon.

I saw improvements in all distances—even my 10-K time went from 35 minutes to 33 minutes.

I was very confident about the Olympic Games in the 1500 meters, and qualified for the Olympic Trials in my first track meet in four years.

The Olympic Boycott in 1980 crushed my spirit for a long time, as it did for so many of us who had waited years to consummate our life's training. The Mardi Gras race was the last competitive marathon I have run to date.

I brought myself to a certain level by changing my training and it worked to a point. But running to the exclusion of all else will make you weak.

Therefore I sought new goals to make myself a better runner and a more complete athlete. I competed in cycling and won the *ABC Superstars* cycling event, and I learned new disciplines such as swimming (something I had never learned as a child) and the martial arts.

Ocean rowing turned out to be the perfect endurance exercise for my arms and shoulders—another form of cardiovascular fitness that is completely opposite of running.

In addition, in the past two years I have worked to put something back into the sport that has given so much to me. I was co-race-director and promoter of the first Los Angeles Pro-Am Marathon in 1980—a race in which we gave away $100,000 in prize money, with women receiving equal prize money for the first time in sports history, and launching professional road-running so that young amateur athletes will have a chance to make money running after the Olympics.

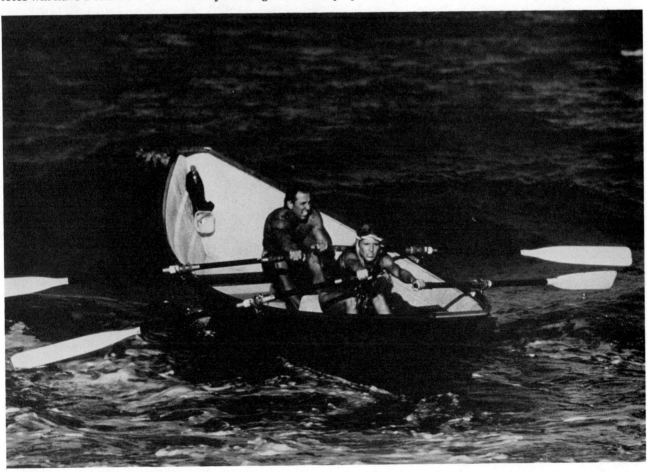

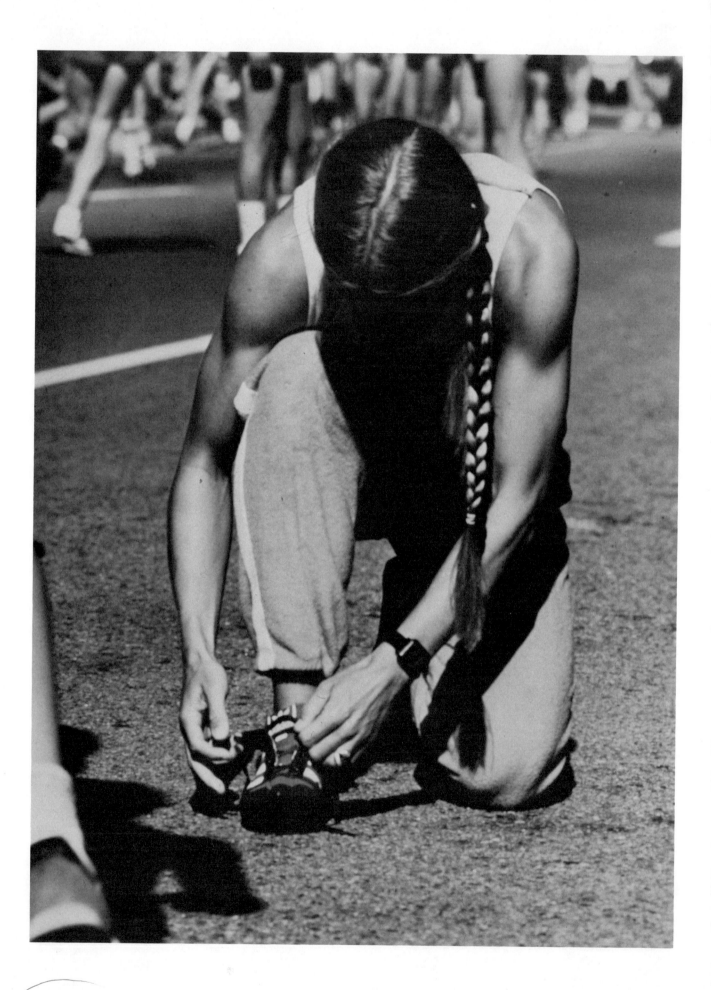

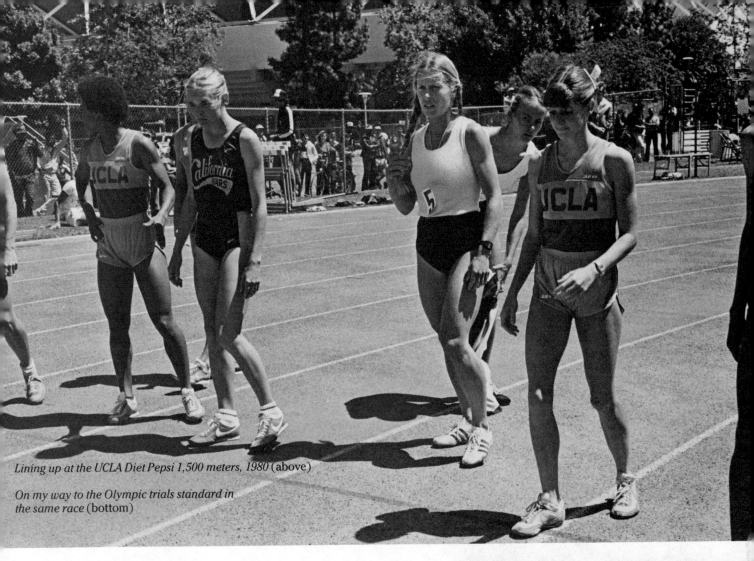

Lining up at the UCLA Diet Pepsi 1,500 meters, 1980 (above)

*On my way to the Olympic trials standard in
the same race* (bottom)

Of course, this book is another way for me to try and turn people
on to fitness and allow them to experience the excitement of getting
fit with the knowledge I've acquired from coaching hundreds of people
over the years, from three-year-olds to pro-football players.

For the first time in Olympic history, there will be a woman's
marathon in 1984. My two-year sabbatical from competition is now
officially over! My greatest challenge waits to be met at the Olympic
Marathon in Los Angeles, 1984. I've decided to go for it once again . . .

This is not just another book on flabby thighs and jelly derrières.
Or how to crawl out of bed every morning and touch your toes a few
times before you hit the road.

I am writing this book because people stop me on the street, in
the supermarket, on airplanes and in restaurants to ask me how to get
fit and get their lives together. They're of all ages and sizes and occu-
pations—from grade fivers to executives and elite athletes. The common thread is that they're all looking for something better for
themselves. To become healthy and as strong as they can be—whatever that means for them, and wherever that takes them.

Sometimes it takes them to the finish line before thousands of
people behind them. And sometimes it takes them only as far as the
starting line. But wherever it takes them, they decided to *Go for It!*

Getting fit and having the energy to pursue your goals is simple.
It's basic, as parts of this book will show you. Some of the exercises,
both mental and physical, might be something you've tried before and

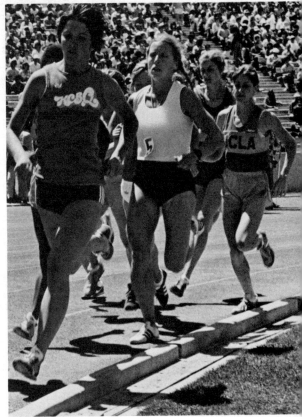

9

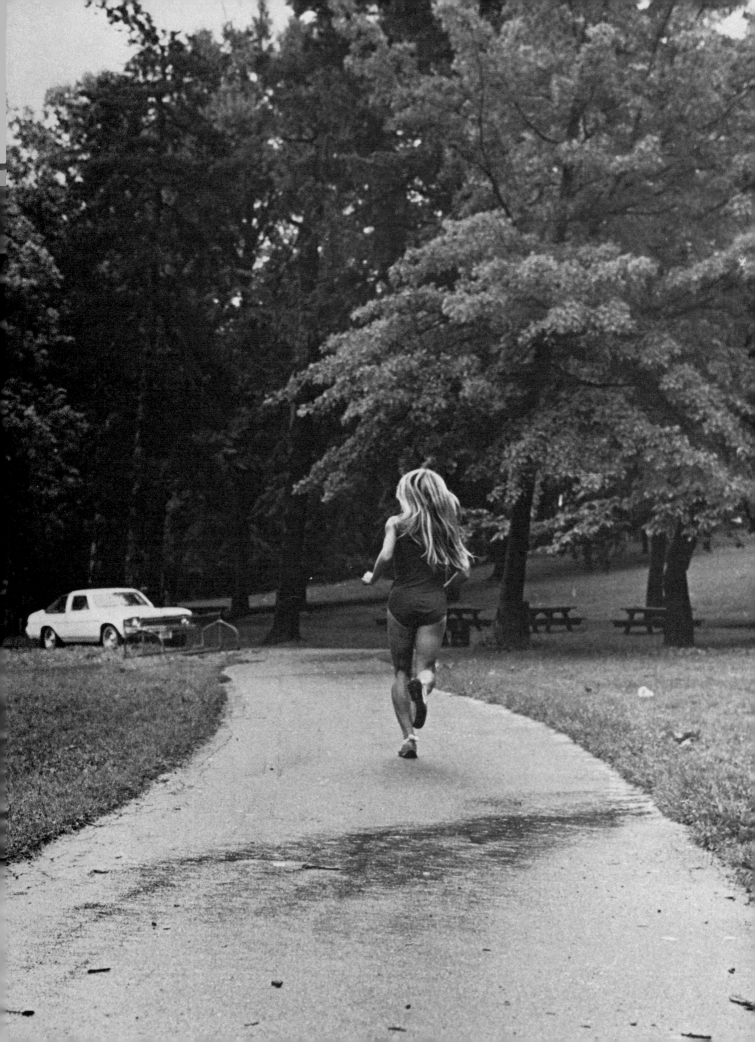

forgotten about. Keep in mind that the muscles respond to exercise for you just as they did for the original Olympians thousands of years ago—and their statues prove it.

I can't promise you your own statue, but I can promise you results if you start these routines today. It may be simple to get in shape, but remember that if it was that easy then everybody would look terrific!

For me, being fit is very special. I still have to wait in line at the supermarket, get stuck on the freeway, and deal with all those other mundane things that simply drain you. The difference for me is that by being fit I can run fifteen miles before breakfast, lift weights, go through the worst endless Monday morning, negotiate in tough business meetings in the afternoon and still have enough energy left after my evening run to give to the ones I love and care for.

That's the payoff. I'm a very lucky person, I've led a charmed life. I've earned it. The payoff is being able to give others my energy.

At one point, though, my life was nothing but chaos. Yet, I was able to pull out great victories for myself. Not everybody is dealt a full deck. The trick is to just play the best you can with the cards you have. Things don't have to be perfect for you to make it.

I live near the Santa Monica Mountains and once or twice a week I run up to the top of these mountains from sea level—a grueling trip that takes me several hours and over 2,000 feet above sea level. My legs and back are strong, but they meet their match fighting gravity all the way up. It's a thirsty trip with no water until the end of the run, and temperatures on a sunny California morning are capable of soaring up to the 90's.

But eventually I get to the top, often not without seeing a lone eagle or deer traveling their home territory.

The view from the top is breathtaking. In one sweep you can see the Pacific Ocean crashing on that sunny beach, the valley plain with the city of Los Angeles magnificently spread out before you, and at the periphery of your vision, the green backs of the other mountains leading to snow-capped peaks only faintly visible above the clouds.

In that majestic silence, I have reflected on the fact that so few people see this view, though the trail is open. You can't drive up—you have to be strong enough to fight the gravity of a 2,000-foot slope to see it.

That made me feel proud to be up there. Privileged to view something so spectacular. Then, a silliness came over me and I waved at an airplane overhead and to everyone else I knew in the world—and everyone I didn't!

Why not? Being fit is fun. Each day belongs to you, and you can successfully conquer it with a winning attitude. It's a great feeling. I know. I want you to know it too. Reading this book is your first step. So, congratulations on wanting more out of life. Now, turn the page and let's *Go for It!*

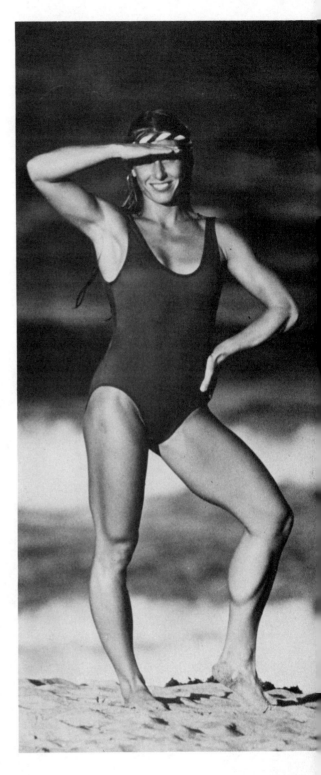

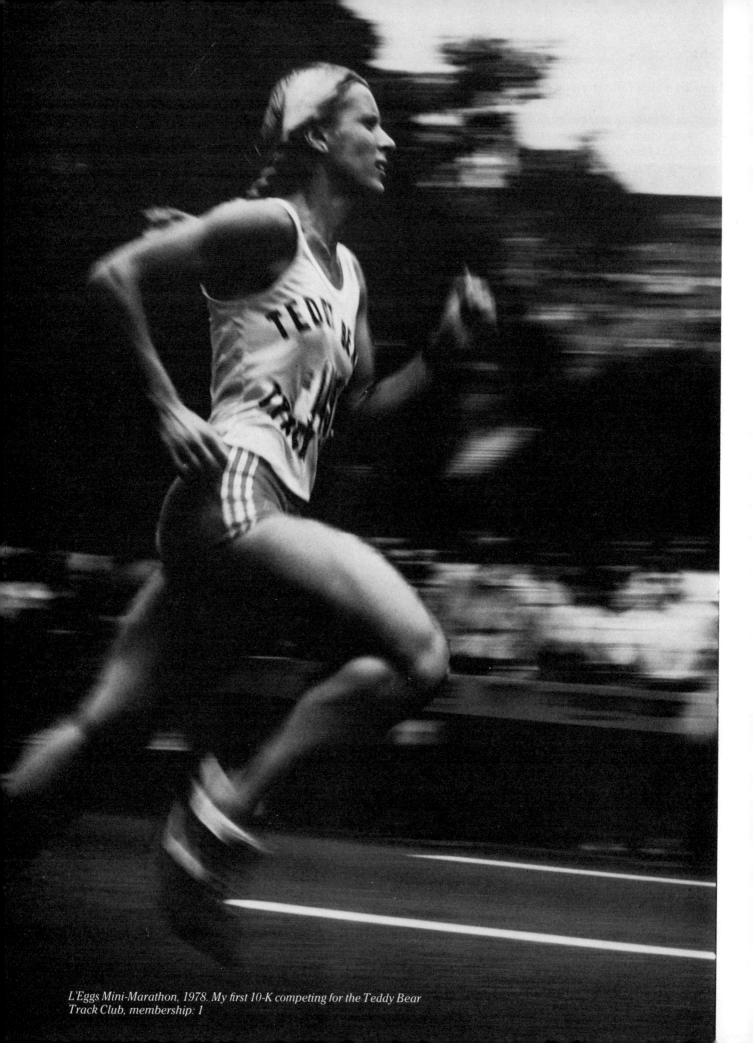

L'Eggs Mini-Marathon, 1978. My first 10-K competing for the Teddy Bear Track Club, membership: 1

1

TEN COMMAND- MENTS FOR SUCCESS

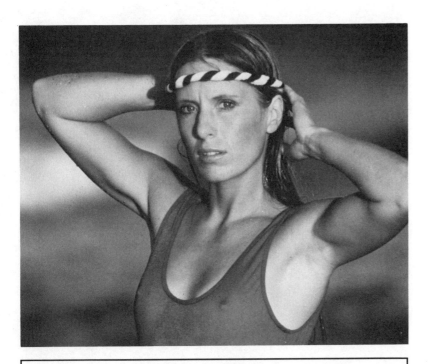

1. **KNOW WHAT YOU WANT**
2. **BE TRUE TO YOURSELF**
3. **STAND TALL AND BE A WINNER**
4. **DISCOVER HOW YOU WANT TO GO FOR IT**
5. **HAVE FUN ALONG THE WAY**
6. **THE BEST STRATEGY IS TO BE PREPARED**
7. **DON'T GET IN YOUR OWN WAY**
8. **TURN YOUR WEAKNESSES TO STRENGTHS**
9. **BECOME WHO YOU ARE**
10. **DON'T SELL OUT**

Commandment Number One: Know What You Want

You've decided to *Go for It*. But what does that mean exactly? What is "it" for you? Is your goal to lose weight or have a million dollars? To fit into your old jeans again or simply be more energetic in the office?

Whatever "it" is for you, write it down. Make a list of your goal in two stages—at six weeks and six months—and post that list in a prominent place. The refrigerator door is a good spot.

Establishing your goals is important, and an example of just how important once came from an unexpected source.

I was running down the street one day when a young man flagged me down, obviously in some distress. He was lost and wanted directions, but didn't even know where he wanted to go. I told him to just keep on driving. After all, if you don't know where you're going, then any road will take you there.

Without a goal, you'll never know when you get there. You must establish where "there" is. And remember, it's *your* goal, *your* dream, and no one else's.

Then hitch your energy onto your dreams and want whatever you want with abundance. I'm willing to bet that you'll surprise yourself.

Commandment Number Two: Be True to Yourself

Now, it's time to make a second list, and this list, I must admit, may be a little more painful than the first one. But believe me, it's every bit as important and it should be posted right next to your list of goals.

Take a piece of paper and write down everything you hate about yourself: perhaps your weight; your laziness; your tendency to procrastinate; the fact that you start but never stick to an exercise program; your mismanagement of money; the way you mistreat people you love; the way you let people you love mistreat you. Write down whatever it is you would like to change, even things that don't relate to a program of fitness. Write them all down and read them every day.

You will find, as the program begins to work, that miraculously some of the items on this list—items that appear to have nothing to do with your goals for fitness at all—will also start to get crossed off. As you begin to take control of your body, you will begin to take control of other parts of your life as well.

For instance, have you ever noticed that you never get sick when you've just fallen in love? Not even so much as a sniffle or blemish. Further, your personality changes magically for the better. You find yourself humming in crowded elevators and ignoring traffic delays because you don't care, you're in love.

However, we all recognize the tenuous quality of love affairs. When it ends, your phone remains silent, you're grouchy, and it feels like you're getting a sore throat.

What I'm talking about here is different. When you *Go for It,* it's a kind of love affair with yourself, with your own body. It can last forever, and with it you will have that same love affair energy that can have you singing in the shower again.

That personal power is available to everyone who achieves his or her goal of better fitness. You will then discover that you are a person who succeeds today in your fitness program; tomorrow in your job; the following day in whatever you wish for.

You are a star—you have the power to make yourself as calm, as fit, as happy as you can be. Seduce yourself!

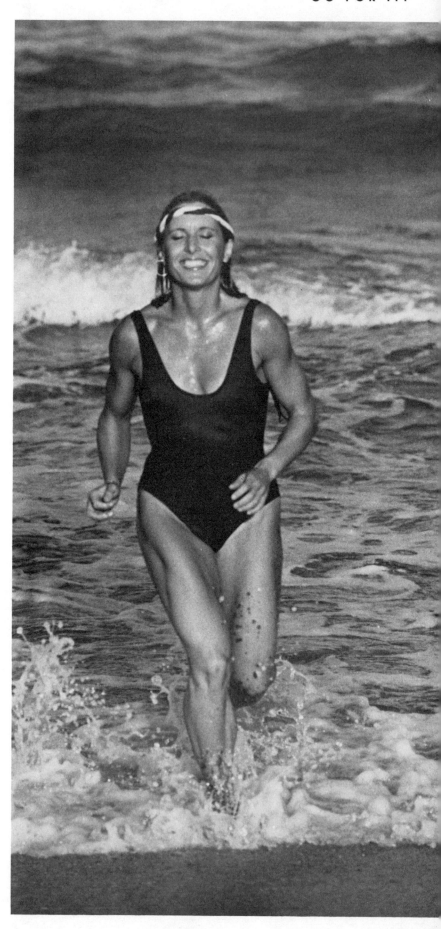

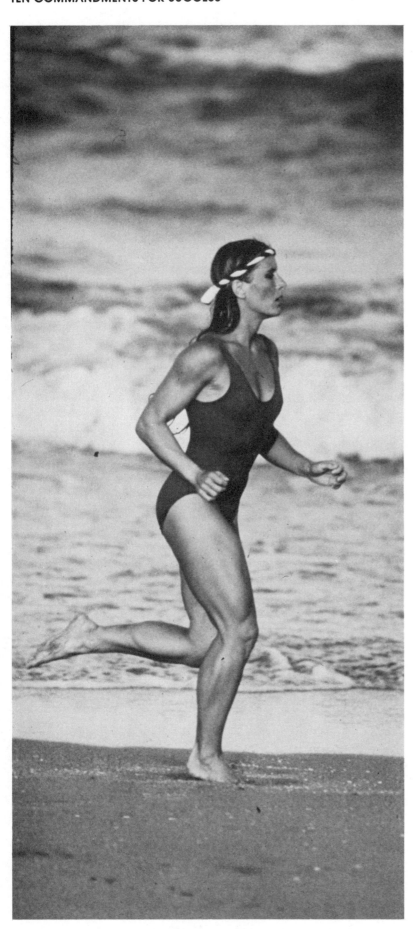

Commandment Number Three: Stand Tall and Be a Winner

Have you ever been in a parade? I was once —the Santa Claus Parade. Crowds of families gathered in anticipation before sunrise, lining the winter streets five deep; even though I was just another snowflake princess, I stood my tallest and smiled my best for each and everyone—but most of all for myself. I knew how excited these kids were to see a real live imaginary snowflake princess, and I didn't want to disappoint them. Now how would it have looked if I had sauntered down the street with my shoulders hunched over and my hands in my pockets? I would have looked terrible, and besides, my eight-pound sequin crown would have fallen off.

Have you ever seen royalty slouch or sag? No. The monarchs of all time hold their heads high and proud even when they're not wearing a crown.

You are unique. Act like royalty and you will be treated like royalty. Don't overdo it— there's a difference between the power of regal posture and the conceited fool with his chest stuck out too far.

Just stand tall, and be a winner.

Commandment Number Four: Discover How You Want to Go for It

Who ever said getting fit can't be fun? Sure, your muscles are going to hurt sometimes (remedies for sore muscles will follow), but the hurt is a good hurt because it means your muscles are growing. Any exercise that is making them grow should be one you enjoy for one simple reason: If you don't enjoy it, you won't stick with it.

I hate to swim. Why? I hate to get my face wet, and I'm not good at it. However, I love to run and that's why it's my main sport activity. When an injury temporarily prevents me from running, I'll use my exercise bicycle or swim the backstroke in the pool so I don't have to get my face wet.

When selecting an activity, don't pooh-pooh skipping rope. It's not only for boxers and school children. There are several new, fancy ropes on the market with ball bearings in the handles and weights on the ropes. It's a lot of fun and you can do it almost anywhere.

Exercise bicycles needn't be dull. Put on some disco, Latin or any other music you prefer and go crazy.

Your exercise plan might include none of the above. Check the "Exercise Chart for Cheaters" (pp. 92–93) for something else that might appeal to you. Whatever it is, know that you are allowed to enjoy it. Remember, if you want to do something big in your life, you have to be willing to try something new.

Commandment Number Five: Have Fun Along the Way

One of the most common questions I am asked at lectures is "How do I know when I've reached the runner's high?" The answer—it's like sex—is when you get there, you'll know about it. There are no signs saying, "You are now entering the ozone layer." You feel good and you know why.

You will discover small pleasures along the way to reaching your ultimate goal of fitness. If you've chosen to exercise by walking, notice what's around you while you walk. Enjoy the smell of the changing seasons, or look forward to meeting people you wouldn't normally meet if you were sitting at home watching TV.

Whatever activity you choose, appreciate all that is happening around you. When you start making better diet choices, don't wait until the exact number of pounds falls off to be happy; enjoy the fact that you are doing something good for yourself. When you retire after a hard day, enjoy the deserved sleep of the person who has decided to go for it.

You will find this new awareness carries over into other parts of your life. You'll be more aware of the moment, more attuned to the present because you have begun to take care of yourself. You are creating your own future, so therefore enjoy every minute that takes you there.

Commandment Number Six: The Best Strategy Is to Be Prepared

At a marathon I ran in Fort Myers, Florida, several years ago, I met a young man on the starting line who asked, "How do you think you are going to do?"

"Just between you and me? I'm going to win," I said. "How about you," I returned. "No idea," he replied. "Hope I can finish."

This was the second marathon I'd ever run in my life. At that moment I was standing in the hottest spot north of the equator: 88 degrees at sunrise, with humidity in the high 90's. By the end of the race, it was 98 degrees with 98 percent humidity, but it didn't matter to me—I had trained in worse and I knew what I could do.

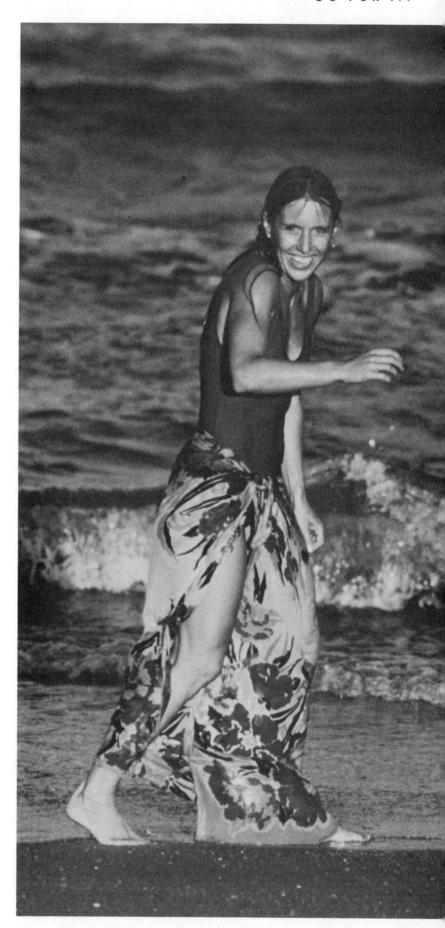

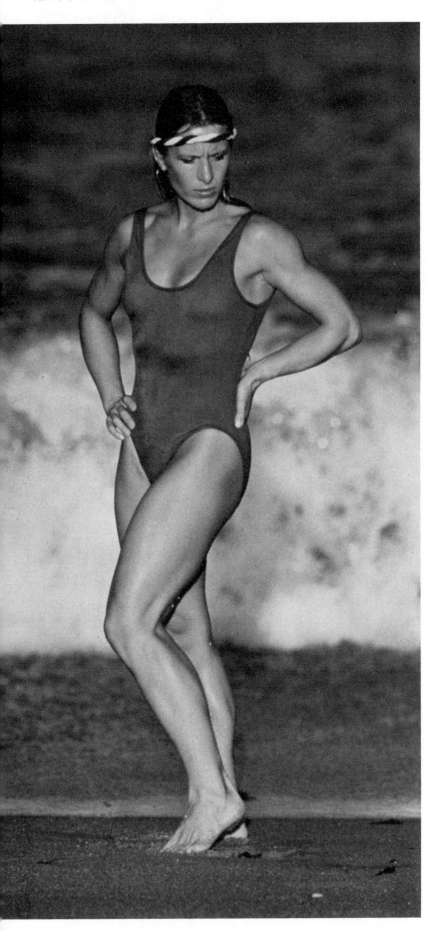

When this fellow caught up with me during the race, he was just about to drop out and forget about his bid to qualify for the Boston Marathon. I encouraged him by saying, "You can do it, just make up your mind you're going to go for it. Shake yourself, and say 'I'm going to do it.'"

He got really excited but his poor preparation for the race made him stop early. My win came after more than a few bleak miles, but with a strong finish: first among the women and ninth among both the men and women in the race.

What I tried to tell him that day and what I want to tell you now is this: Give it your best shot by believing you are a winner, and don't wait until you get to the starting line to do it.

Be realistic—you don't prepare for Wimbledon the day before the tennis tournament begins. The preparation starts months, even years before the big event. It's desire plus action that equals success.

You deserve the best. Believe in yourself enough to give it your best, and you'll be a winner no matter what the final score is.

Commandment Number Seven: Don't Get in Your Own Way

Observing athletes preparing for their moment of truth has always been fascinating to me.

As a sprinter, I, like the others, had my little rituals I performed each time to help relieve tension. I always took off my sweatsuits and folded them very neatly one by one before getting into the blocks.

But after a time, in reaction to the mounting pressure I began to create for myself, I became more and more fastidious in this folding and straightening.

Each new adjustment failed to relieve the nervous wreck I was becoming with this superstitious ritual until one day the start official actually called me for delaying the race.

And so, over the years, I've developed a technique which I call "Garbage In, Garbage Out." It's sort of a "There I go again" realization that stops the continuation of negative thoughts or actions, and turns them into positive thoughts and actions. It works like this. Sometimes in the middle of a marathon, I actually start laughing out loud at some of the things that go through my head. For instance, the gun goes off, and after thirty seconds into the marathon I've looked at my chronograph and said to myself, "Oh gee—only thirty seconds gone by, and I'm already dead." So I laugh and say to myself, "This is just garbage in, garbage out," and keep going. Now some of my best races have started out like this—and so have some of my worst. The difference is that in the victories, I have been able to laugh at myself and use this commandment for success to fulfill my potential and go on to triumph.

You can too. Say, for instance, you're trying to lift a weight. You've already got it up to your shoulders when that voice inside your head says: "Gee, this is heavy." This qualifies as a garbage in, garbage out thought. If you don't get rid of it, that little demon voice will soon say something else like "And besides this weight being heavy, boy, am I tired today . . ." So at the first whimper, squelch it by saying "garbage in, garbage out" or your equivalent.

But the weight is still only at your shoulders. Now what? Have you forgotten "Commandment for Success Number 8"? Turn your weakness into strength.

Use your imagination. In my mind's eye, I picture myself lifting two great spheres of light—the sun and the moon on each end of the bar, with my legs astride the earth. I lift the sun and the moon up to the sky. In this way, I not only garbage out that weak thought, I obliterate it with the colossal image of myself lifting two parts of the sky to the heavens.

I've shared with you my secret image. Now, make up your own and store it for the times of need. Create an image of yourself being powerful and strong. This image should appear at the first peep of that little voice trying to introduce a barrier between who you are and who you want to become.

Your image can be anything you want. If you're swimming your second lap and beginning to tire, imagine yourself in the middle of a world class swimming competition ahead of the Mark Spitzes and Tracy Caulkinses. If you'd rather not do that last lap around the track, imagine yourself at the front of 500 marathoners with the closest person behind you 10 feet away.

Remember, it's your fantasy image. Make it as classy as you want: It works.

Commandment Number Eight: Turn Your Weaknesses to Strengths

The successful person in sports or in a career does not use alibis when he or she is not doing well. Rather, he or she analyzes the weakness and acts to improve it.

For example, if you're a gymnast who needs work on the fluidity or smoothness of the routine, think carefully of the problem areas.

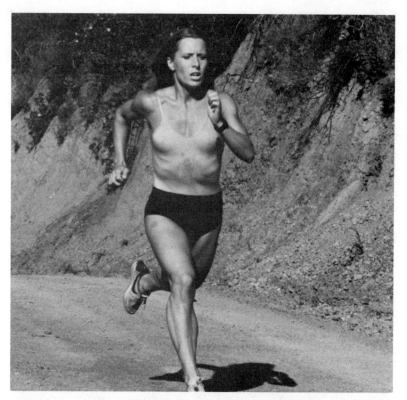

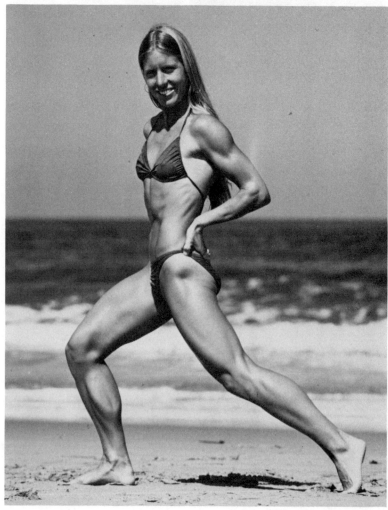

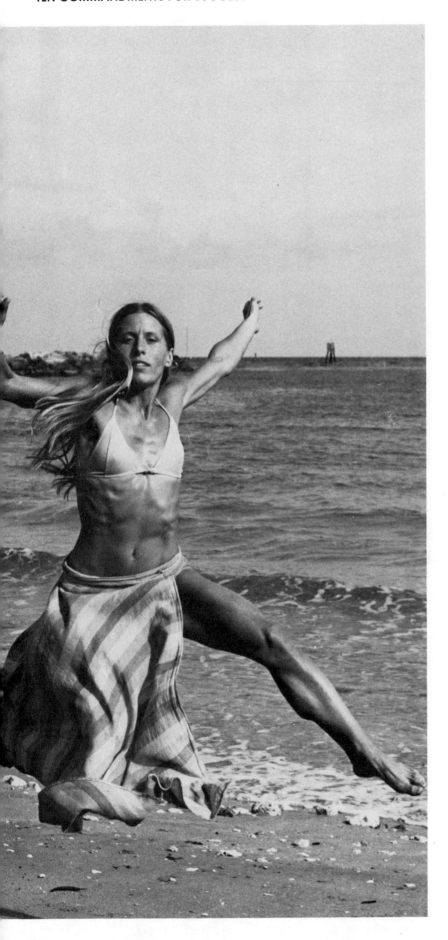

Areas to review might be your transitions from one pose to another, the music you're using, or your lack of stamina causing difficulty with the end of the routine. By working on one aspect of the whole problem, you will progress to mastering the weaknesses.

One winter I decided that, if nothing else, I would learn to run keeping my arms tucked in instead of waving from side to side. I wrote on an index card "ARMS," covered it with plastic and sewed it on to the sleeve of my windbreaker. The ink faded and the plastic cracked, but even the rustle of that tag in the wind made me think of keeping my arms tucked in. The results were recognized by a photographer doing a photo study on my running form. He commented, "Gayle, your form is book perfect, especially your arms. You must really be happy to come by all this naturally." I just laughed and thought of my list.

You see, it works. Know what your weaknesses are, list the ways you know how to conquer them, and go to it. Your weaknesses will then become your strengths.

Commandment Number Nine: Become Who You Are

As you establish your goals and begin to reach them, you will, by definition, become different; different from who you were before you made the decision to change your life; different from the people who chose not to make that decision; different from the people who don't know what your goals are; different from the people who aren't motivated like you; different from the people who prefer to believe they aren't responsible for their own lives.

I recently ran into an old hometown acquaintance I had not seen in many years. He had kept up with me through my athletic career by reading in newspapers and sports magazines.

"Well, I must say, Gayle, success is very becoming to you," he said. "But we always knew you were different."

He was right. I was different and not ashamed of it either. In high school, I was the laughingstock of the class when they saw me outside one day, running in a snowstorm wearing a shower cap. It didn't faze me in the least. Realizing I was different was my first step to success.

Being different and proud could well be your step to success, too. Think about it; when you see what passes for normal on the street, aren't you glad you're different? To become who you are, you must be unique.

Accept it. Rejoice in it. How many people in this world are living their dreams?

Be glad you are not one of the throng! And don't believe for one minute that it's too crowded at the top. There's plenty of room at the top. You and I both know that it's at the bottom where it's crowded.

Commandment Number Ten: Don't Sell Out

In our headlong rush to "get there," it's easy to close our senses to the beauty of just "being there," of taking time to feel pleasure in our decisions about ourselves. What has beauty got to do with success? Everything. Because not to notice the beauty of life is to fail at living.

But you and I know that life doesn't always deal you a perfect hand. The trick is to realize that and to make the best of it. At times, though, the burden of our situation can be so heavy that at the moment it seems too unbearable to think that anything good can come from it without seriously compromising yourself. As you'll learn in the exercise section, if you lug around a weight long enough, eventually you get stronger—there's no need to sell out.

When I first became one of the top five marathon runners in the world, it only took a few hours until it seemed as if the whole world wanted me for something—an interview, a race, an appearance, an endorsement. I'll never forget a follow-up meeting to one of these calls which was held in the boardroom of a large soft drink company. Picture a lavish room with a lot of cigar smoke. The interchange was brief—they wanted me to endorse their diet drink and I refused, stating carcinogenic ingredients as the reason. They offered me six figures as payment. I refused—I don't and won't drink the stuff.

The chairman of the board was turning red with exasperation. He then cited examples of young tennis stars barely out of braces endorsing similar products. It made no impression on me. I've always thought that many people feel no responsibility to their celebrity status. Celebrity is awarded to you by the people who follow you. It's an admiration, a respect that is conferred, and there is a moral issue at hand—to endorse good products for instance. If your kid has ever wailed in the supermarket when he can't have that sugar-and-chemical-laden cereal with the current hero's face on it, then you know what I'm talking about.

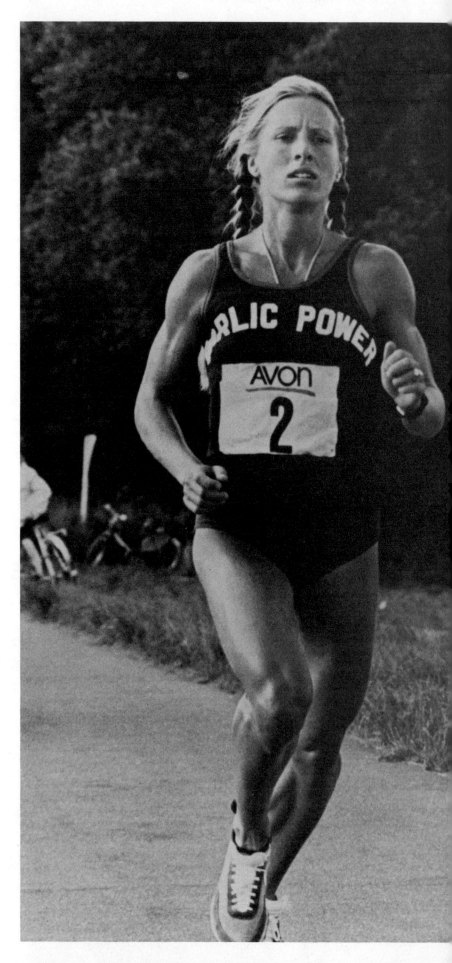

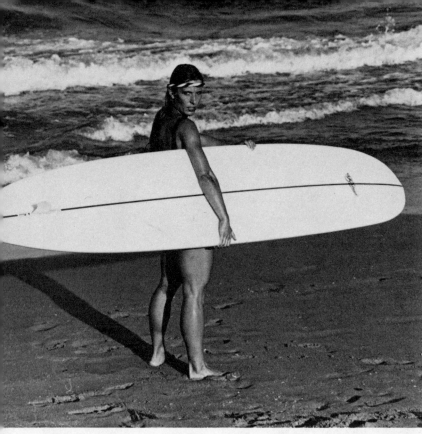

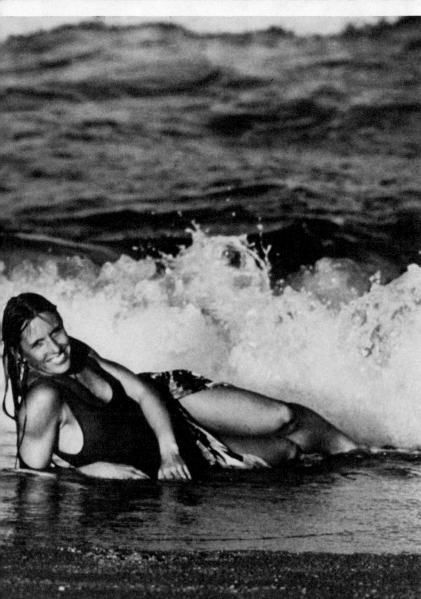

At any rate, I left the diet drink people feeling drained. At that point, nothing seemed to be going right. I returned home and realized how broke I really was. The electricity had been cut off and so had the telephone. I began rising at sunrise and going to bed at sunset in order to make best use of the daylight. Cold showers were the order of the day, but I was determined to keep on training for the World Championships in Germany. Luckily in the tropics, you can always pick fruit somewhere, and as I became thinner, the hungriness made me faster and tougher.

Fortunately, the organizers of the race paid my fare overseas. The night before the marathon I thought of the diet drink company and all the other similar sponsors' names that would be on my competitors' jerseys. What could I put on my shirt that I believed in? Hastily I sewed GARLIC POWER on my shirt.

Where is the beauty in all this? I'd love to write the perfect Hollywood ending, saying that even though I hadn't eaten in three days, I won the race and got a world record. That's not what happened. I didn't win the race, but even though I had lost the battle that day, I felt closer to winning the war when a little German girl came up to me afterward. She wanted to know what my shirt said. I translated it for her and she asked me if I ate garlic and if I thought it was good for you if you wanted to be an athlete someday.

I looked her right in the eye and said yes, leaned down, and gave her a big hug. The beauty of that truth meant a great deal to me at that moment. I felt a personal triumph that erased the pain of the marathon. I hadn't sold out.

You can't win *all* the time. And while the losses can be painful (let's face it, nobody *likes* to lose), I want you to know that it happens to me, too—there's no shame in losing if you've given it your best shot. Also keep in mind that there's no dignity in reaching the top if you had to sell out to get there.

Go out and look at the stars tonight. Yours is up there someplace, waiting just for you. Life is beautiful—have fun and enjoy its variety. Enjoy the wonder of the small surprises that come from setting your own standards and sticking to them.

Success is out there waiting for you, just like the stars in the sky. You just have to look up there and see it.

It looks great, doesn't it?

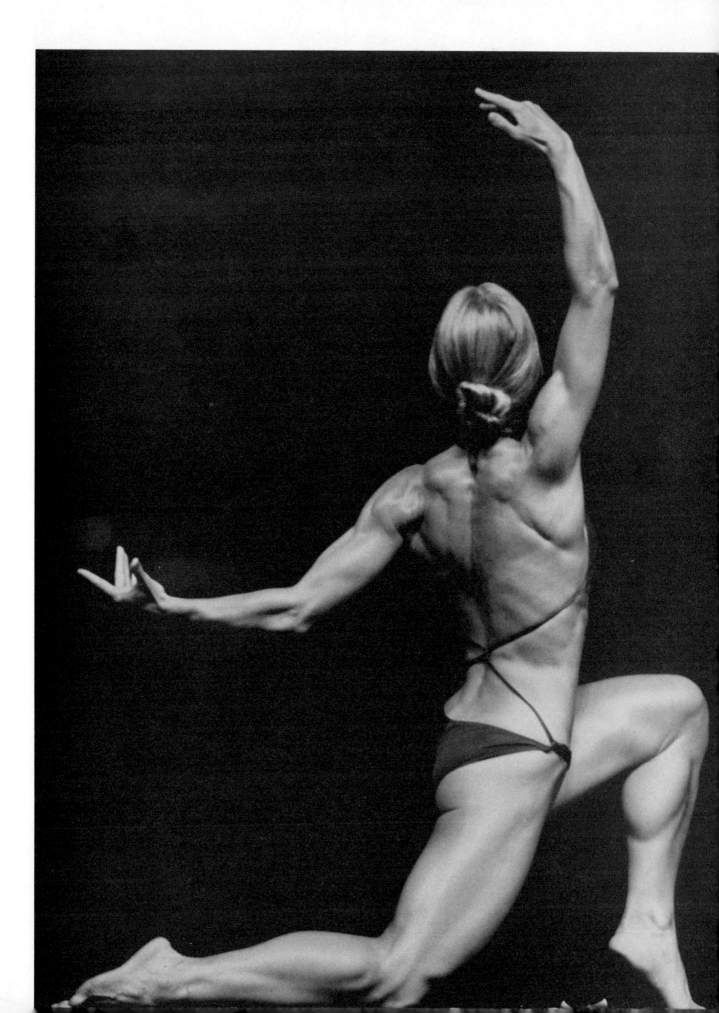

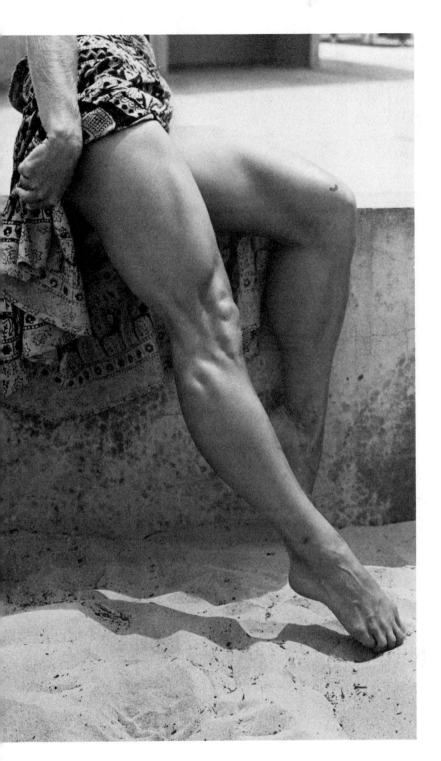

13 Ways to Make Sure You Don't Go for It

This is the last list contained in these ten rules to success, and I've already filled this list out for you. All you have to do is post it in the same place as the other two.

This list is an accumulation of negative attitudes I've noticed by people who constantly fail in their attempts to get fit. The items reflect the attitudes that act as barriers between who you are and who you want to become. For the person who keeps putting off the fitness program, this list of don't's will serve as a constant reminder of the habits that are sure to sabotage even the best game plan for fitness.

1. Eat when you're depressed.
2. Blame your glands, metabolism or genetics when you gain another fifteen pounds. ("Everyone in my family is fat.")
3. Make up for the depression you feel about being out of shape by going on an eating binge.
4. Cancel a date with someone you'd like to know better because you feel too fat and ugly.
5. Start buying baggy clothes and convince yourself it's because they are more comfortable.
6. Buy food as a special reward for good behavior before the good behavior.
7. When your lover says he/she likes you better heavier, believe it.
8. Feel sorry for yourself because you don't have time to get in shape.
9. Eat heavily before you exercise; then convince yourself it's bad for you to exercise after a big meal.
10. Eat like a pig on Sunday night because you start your diet on Monday morning. Then, don't.
11. Persuade yourself it will be easier to get in shape when it's summertime.
12. When summer comes, see Number 1.
13. Never give it your best shot, so you'll always have a good excuse.

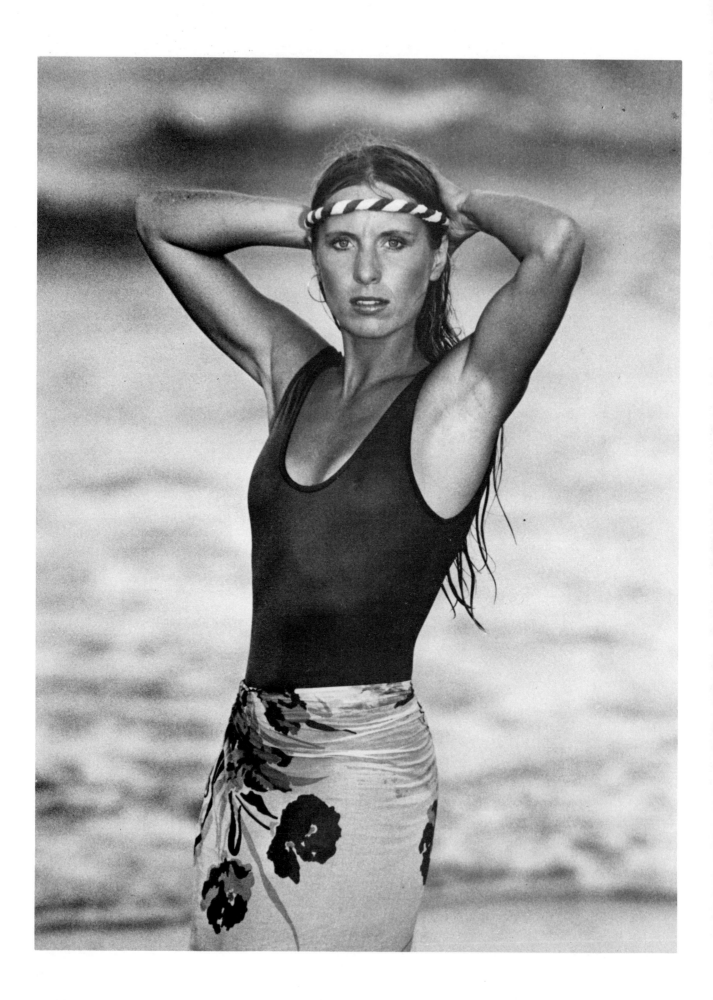

2

HOW TO GO FOR IT —EXERCISES

HOW TO GO FOR IT

If you have lain there like a canvas all your life, waiting for that magic person to paint a fantasy on it for you—forget it. Now is the time to paint your *own* canvas.

It's a tragedy that so few people ever really learn to be as strong and alive as they can be. Why live a half-life, always feeling too tired to cope? Socrates, the famous philosopher of the ancient Greeks, said, "No person has the right to be an amateur in the matter of physical fitness. What a disgrace it is for a man to grow without ever seeing the beauty and strength of which his body is capable."

Getting stronger is not only important for athletes. Let's face it— it's the little things in life that count, and if you're a woman who's ever had to wait for a man to come and open the pickle jar for you, you know what I'm talking about.

Muscular strength and sculpting a new shape for your body is exciting and fulfilling, and it doesn't matter whether you are rich or poor, tall or short, female or male. At the times in my life when I've been poorest, I was living on a skateboard budget; but running down the street, my body was handling like a finely tuned Porsche.

Everyone can get stronger, and every time you do something for yourself in the fitness department, it is an investment in your future. The effects of a lifetime of fitness are cumulative—like money in the bank, like savings you work for in your twenties, thirties and forties and accumulate so that you can enjoy your seventies, eighties and nineties. Just as the money you've already saved is still in the bank even if you temporarily stop saving, should you happen to fall out of a fitness plan for a week, a month, or even a year, your body retains memory of the route to fitness, and you have only to guide it back. The return trip is much quicker than the original journey.

The state of the economy, pollution and the actions of other people are all things over which we have little or no control. We all have a need to feel good about ourselves, and having physical control over the strength and energy of your own body is something that no one can take away from you. It can't be taxed. It belongs to no one but you. And as the world moves toward harder times, this precious self-mastering takes on increasing significance. In the chaos that is happening around us, we need at least to be in complete physical command of ourselves—to have the strength to cope, to remain rational and to retain positive values. This is to have achieved personal freedom.

Vic Boff, one of the world's pioneers in physical fitness, has said, "Always remember—the care of one's body is a sacred responsibility —the first you accept and the last you lay down."

Go for It!—let's begin.

THE BEAUTY OF USING YOUR OWN BODY WEIGHT

It is not always essential to lift weights in order to be strong and have a sleek physique. You may not live near a spa or gym or a place where you can readily purchase some dumbbells right away. That's OK. It doesn't mean that you can't start, because you always have your own body weight to use.

Chin-ups, pull-ups, sit-ups and push-ups are all excellent muscle stimulants, and you can do them in the privacy of your own living room. Even if you have access to dumbbells, you can do exercises using your own body weight as a change, or when you're traveling or on vacation. Put some upbeat music on and let yourself go.

Learning to balance and exert your muscles using your own body weight is also a marvelous way to feel your own energy. Just ask any dancer or gymnast—possessors of some of the world's most sensual physiques.

DUMBBELLS, ANKLE WEIGHTS AND CHINNING BARS

These items offer resistance needed to get you stronger and shape your body. They are available at most sporting goods stores and department stores, and are a reasonable investment—certainly a fraction of the expense of joining a health spa.

Classified ads in the newspaper are another place to look for used dumbbells—they never wear out, and a coat of paint in your favorite color can give you a color-coordinated look.

Telephone books, plastic milk jugs filled with water, or even unopened cans of food can be used as dumbbells, but I personally find it difficult to get motivated to work out using a telephone book. And as far as the other items are concerned, there are disadvantages—suppose someone ate the can of beans you had been using all week for your workout? Make a commitment and buy some dumbbells and ankle weights. After all, you're in the big time now.

USING A MIRROR

An important point to remember when exercising is to concentrate on the muscle you're working on. It's hard to do that when you're staring at the wall. To insure concentration, use a mirror. Look at the muscle you are using. Appreciate the strength and beauty of it while working through the movement. Watch the shape of it change as it contracts and extends, and you'll also be sure of perfect form as well.

SHAPE OR STRENGTH?

There is a difference. If you perform the exercise many times (fifteen to twenty reps) with a light weight, you will shape the muscle. To achieve strength, you must lift a relatively heavier weight fewer times. If power is your aim, then use a weight which can only be lifted three to five times. However, don't lose your form for any number of repetitions—as good form is most of the magic in getting stronger. A realistic goal for general fitness is to aim for three sets of the exercise with ten to twelve repetitions in each set.

ANATOMY OF SUCCESSFUL FITNESS

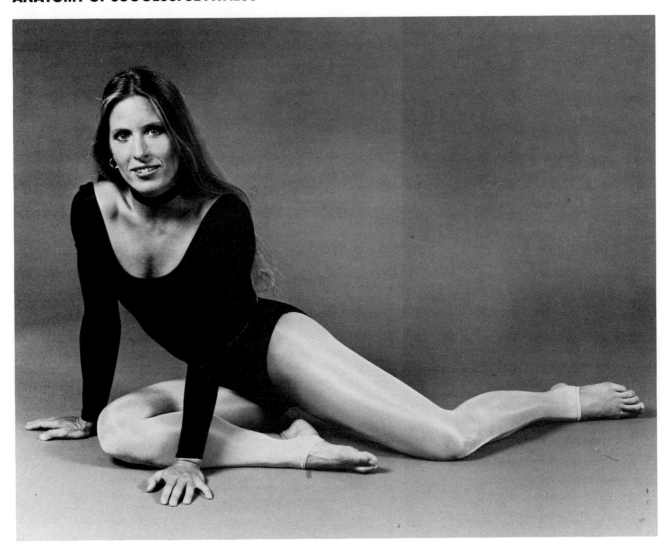

People often ask me: "Why should I exercise?" Exercising and doing things to stay healthy is sort of like paying rent. You can do other things first with your money of course, but, eventually, if you don't take care of yourself you won't have any place to live.

ATTENTION BEGINNERS

Because you're beginning, remember that it's important to start off realistically. For example, if you've never done a bent-knee sit-up before, it's better to start with two and work up to ten rather than start off with ten the first day. By overdoing it because of initial enthusiasm, you may be only able to do four the next day. I've seen even elite athletes coming back after time off overdo it on their first day. People get so gung-ho the first day that they strain themselves and never continue.

At the same time, you have to *try hard.* Not used to "paying the rent," as it were, your muscles may feel some ache. That's good. The first few days are for learning about your body and its limits. There is no "right" number of times to repeat each exercise, only what's right for you. Try hard and *Go for It!*

ON SLEEPING AND EATING—A FEW TIPS

- Don't eat late at night before sleep.

- Don't eat a big meal when you're really tired.

- Sleep is as important as the training. Catch afternoon naps whenever possible. Even if you don't sleep, twenty minutes of complete relaxation lying down will refresh you for the evening workout. Ironically, the more you train, the more fitfully you sometimes sleep at night. The body is too exhausted to sleep. Listen to your body—it always tries to do the best thing for you. Naps help prevent the cycle of fatigue, which destroys your body, tearing down rather than building.

So take care of yourself.

BREATHING

Never hold your breath when lifting weights or doing an exercise.

Remember
    exhale during the exertion phase

    inhale during the return to the start position

EXAMPLE—Sit-ups
- Take in a deep breath when you're ready to start
- Breathe *out* when bringing the trunk toward the knees
- Breathe *in* when returning to start position

Any of these exercises can be made more or less difficult depending upon the number of repetitions, the weight used and the effort applied.

STRETCHING

A good stretch—it satisfies like the savory intensity of a big yawn. Animals know this instinctively. Ever watch a cat arch her back and stretch after a nap?

Unfortunately, we tend to ignore our instincts to stretch and this can be very dangerous for an athlete. Stretching helps to prevent injuries. Stretching is also an inseparable ingredient of speed. Remember that a relaxed muscle that has been stretched is capable of a more forceful contraction and therefore more strength, the result of which is more speed. Think of a bow and arrow: The farther you can stretch back the string, the faster and farther the arrow can travel when it's released.

In addition, stretching improves circulation in the muscle, bringing fresh oxygen to a muscle which may have been worked momentarily to exhaustion. Stretching the worked muscle between sets of an exercise, for instance, can allow you to do more work with that muscle.

IMPORTANT

• Never bounce when stretching

• Never force to pain

• Hold each position to a slow count of 30

• Use stretching as part of your warm-up and cool-down, especially for aerobic activity

---

STOMACH

We call it our stomach, tummy, paunch, belly, gut or corporation, but the shape it's in is directly related to the muscles of the abdomen and the presence or absence of the fat that covers them.

Erect posture is impossible without tonicity in this area. Injury to the back and legs is greater when there is softness in the abdomen, and there is not an athletic sport that does not use the abdominal muscles. Also, abdominal strength is necessary for strength in the low back, which is the source of power in the human body.

These exercises are as tough as you need them—they've worked for me and hundreds of athletes I've coached. Sleek stomachs are sexy. Follow the directions and find out for yourself.

ADVICE TO BEGINNERS

If you've never done a bent-knee sit-up before, remember it is better to start with 2 and work up to 10 than be too ambitious and do 10 sit-ups the first day. By overdoing it, you may find that the next day you can only do 4; or worse, that you can't do any because you are too sore.

If you find on the first day that you can't do even 1, then establish 1 as your initial goal. Keep trying every day until you can do that 1 sit-up. Then try for 2, and so on, remembering there is no "right" number of times to repeat each exercise—only what's right for you.

On the other hand, don't be *too* easy on yourself. Try hard and *Go for It.*

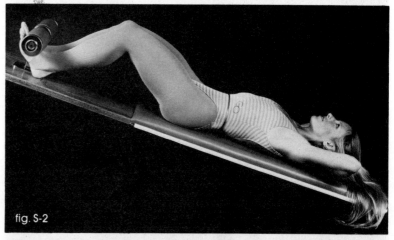

fig. S-1

fig. S-2

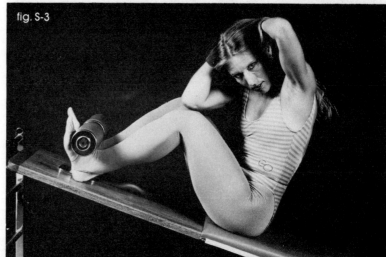

fig. S-3

Knee to Chest

Starting Position: Lie on your back with your legs out straight, feet together. Press the small of your back against the floor. (Ask a friend to try to slip a piece of paper under your back. If you are doing it right, your friend cannot slide the paper under there.)
Movement: Bring both knees up to your chest and lower them again, unbending as you go, until you reach the starting position. Don't let your feet touch the floor. Repeat the exercise, building some momentum as you go. When you can do 50 of these, you're ready to do the same exercise with 1 lb.–5 lb. ankle weights.
Goal: Beginners 25, Advanced 50.
(*fig. S-1*)

Bent-Knee Sit-ups

Bent-knee sit-ups are harder than the regular kind, but a faster and more effective cure for midriff bulge.
Note: Always do sit-ups with bent knees. *Do not* hook your feet under the sofa or china cabinet, or have a friend sit on them. You won't really be using the stomach muscles to pull yourself up, but will instead be putting strain on the wrong muscle—the psoas muscle next to your groin.*
Starting Position: Lie on your back with your hands behind your head and draw your knees up, your feet flat on the floor.
Movement: Think of curling your spine as you lift your torso until your elbows touch your knees. Return to starting position for a brief second (just to touch your back to the floor), and repeat.
Goal: Beginners 25, Advanced 50.
(*figs. S-2 and 3*)

* Figures S-2 and 3 show sit-ups on a slant board—a more difficult variation, and the only time the feet should be secured when doing sit-ups.

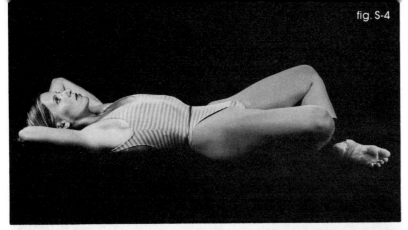

fig. S-4

Crunches

Starting Position: Lie on your back, hands behind your head, legs crossed Indian style. Press the small of your back flat against the floor. (Remember the paper test?)
Movement: Raise your head as far as possible and hold that crunched-up position for 2 counts. (I say "one steamboat, two steamboats," but be as creative as you wish.) Repeat this routine until you feel a burning sensation in your stomach muscles. Then do 5 more. Remember to keep your back pressed against the floor. That gives the best results.
Goal: Beginners 25, Advanced 50.
(*figs. S-4 and 5*)

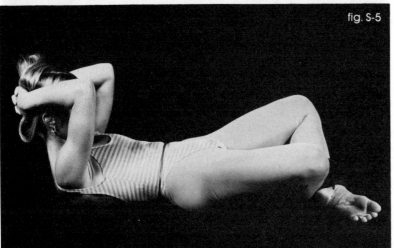

fig. S-5

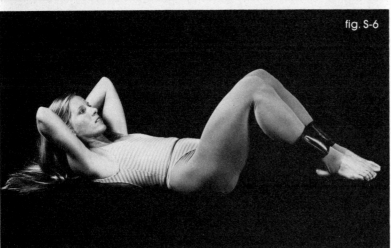

fig. S-6

Cradle Crunches

Starting Position: Lie on the floor, hands behind your head, the small of your back pressed flat against the floor. Bend your knees up as far as possible with your feet 1 inch off the floor.
Movement: Raise up your trunk as far as possible and exhale (really exhale) and hold for 2 counts. Then, inhale (really inhale) as you return to the starting position. When it feels like your stomach muscles are catching on fire, hold the starting position for 50 counts.
Goal: Beginners 10, Advanced 25.
(*fig. S-6*)

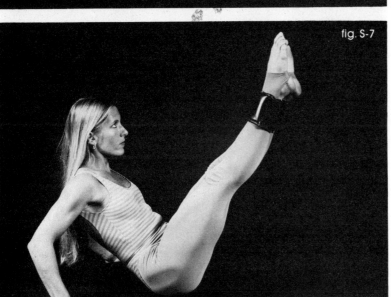

fig. S-7

Jackknife with Ankle Weights

Purpose: Uses upper and lower abdomen.
Starting Position: Sit on floor, legs together and in front of you. Hands beside you on floor for support.
Movement: Keeping legs together, bring feet off floor. Bring legs into a V position. Pause and lower legs. Repeat.
Goal: Beginners 10, Advanced 25.
(*fig. S-7*)

Bench Crunches

Purpose: Uses upper abdomen.
Starting Position: Lie on floor with your legs up on a bench or chair. Hands behind neck.
Movement: Curl your trunk up while exhaling. Return to starting position and repeat.
Goal: Beginners 25, Advanced 50.
(*figs. S-8 and 9*)

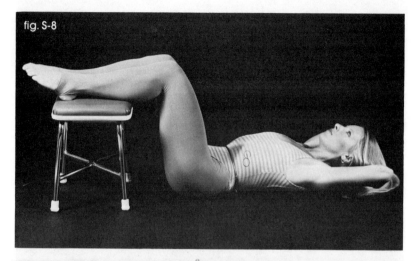

fig. S-8

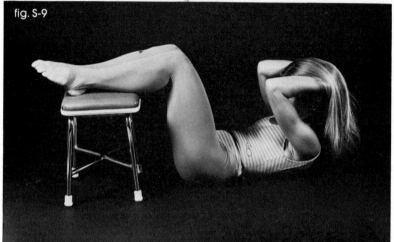

fig. S-9

Cobra Stretch

Purpose: After all that work on your muscles, this exercise is an absolute *must.* When you work your muscles, they contract and you need to stretch them afterward. Stretching increases flexibility, which is important for strength, and helps prevent injury.
Starting Position: Lie on your stomach with your hands directly under your chest, fingers touching.
Movement: Raise your trunk slowly, mouth open, looking up. Hold for a 50 count.
(*fig. S-10*)

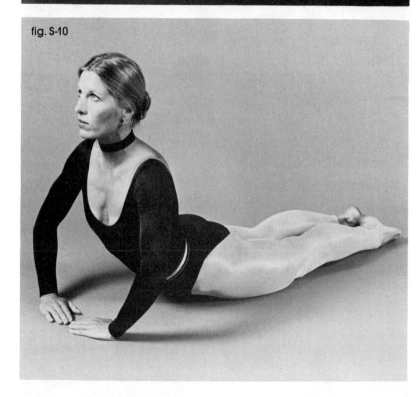

fig. S-10

DERRIÈRE

Your derrière needs more exercise than it gets from sitting on a chair. Even in the leanest athlete, it is still nearly always the fleshiest part of the body. The fat is covering the large gluteus maximus muscles for protection of the lower spine and also for insulation and plain old comfort. Clearly, some people have provided for more "comfort" in this area than is necessary or even healthful!

The "glutes" are the major muscles in the lower spine, and are the movers in lower trunk and hip movement and in all knee bending movements, ranging from climbing stairs, running and skiing to skipping rope, cycling and dancing. These muscles rotate the thigh outward, so that lateral movements in tennis, racquetball and football, for instance, all rely on the strength of the glutes and the hip flexor muscles.

Aesthetically, a droopy derrière is never in style, and it even affects the way you walk.

North American soldiers sent overseas in World War I and World War II were amazed and fascinated by the walk of the Italian and French women. What they were actually viewing was the movement of developed gluteus maximus muscles: an action they found to be incredibly sexy. Gina Lollobrigida and Brigitte Bardot are two of the many screen stars who used this type of walk—although I doubt if even *one* movie magazine ever gave the gluteus muscles any credit for it!

You may also be interested to know that in the *Book of Lists* by Irving Wallace, *et al.,* "small buns" were listed by women as the top priority in physical appeal of men. Biceps, which men felt were a top attraction for women, didn't even make top ten as far as women were concerned.

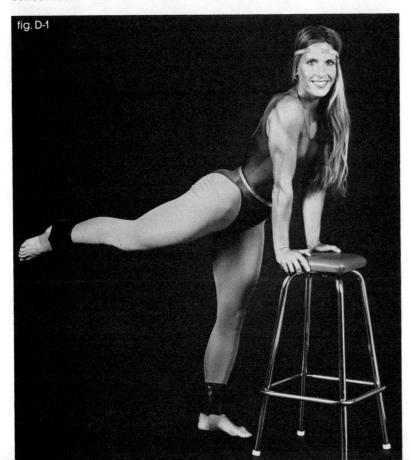

fig. D-1

Back Kick with Ankle Weights

Purpose: Uses buttocks and hips.
Starting Position: Stand erect, holding on to the back of chair as shown.
Movement: Move one leg back slowly as shown. Pause. Return to start position and repeat for desired number of repetitions. Switch legs.
Goal: Beginners 25, Advanced 50.
(*fig. D-1*)

Side Leg Raises with Ankle Weights

Purpose: Uses buttocks, hip and lower abdomen.
Starting Position: Lie on floor on your side as shown.
Movement: Raise up your leg sideways as wide as possible. Lower and repeat for desired number of repetitions. Switch legs.
Goal: Beginners 25, Advanced 50.
(*figs. D-2 and 3*)

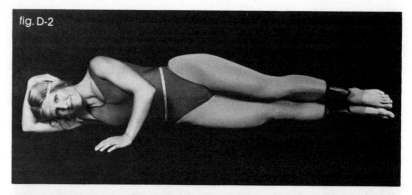

fig. D-2

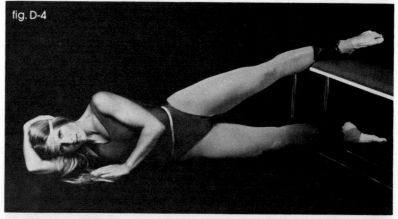

fig. D-3

Lying Side Scissor with Bench

Purpose: Uses buttocks, hip and lower abdomen.
Starting Position: Lie on your side with one foot up on bench as shown.
Movement: Keeping both knees locked, move the bottom leg up and down rapidly. Your moving foot should not touch the floor once you begin. Switch legs.
Goal: Beginners 25, Advanced 50.
(*figs. D-4 and 5*)

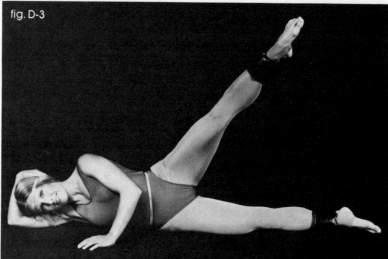

fig. D-4

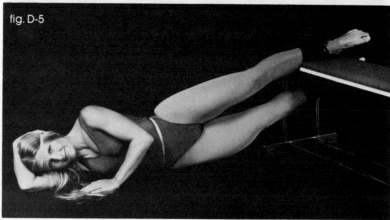

fig. D-5

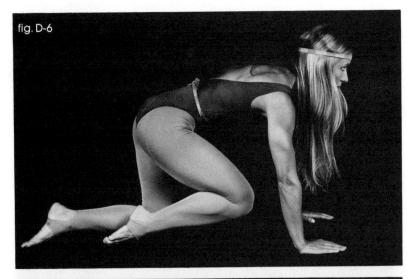

fig. D-6

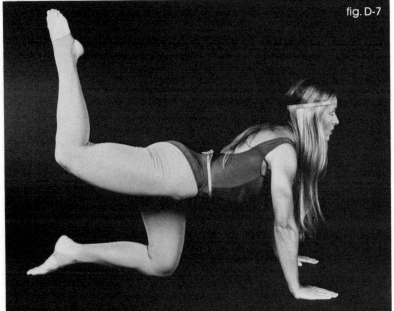

fig. D-7

Kick Backs

Purpose: Uses buttocks and hamstring muscle where it connects with buttocks.
Starting Position: On all fours, hands shoulder width, back straight.
Movement: Bring knee to chest, then kick leg straight back, sweeping foot high into the air. Return to start position and repeat.
Goal: Beginners 25, Advanced 50.
(*figs. D-6 and 7*)

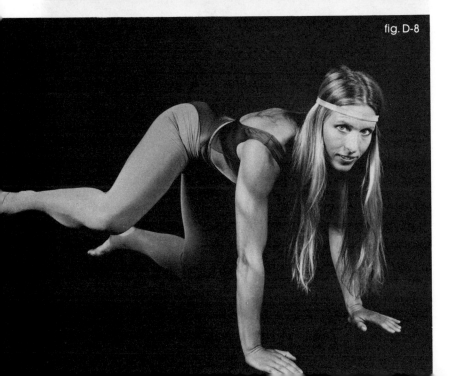

fig. D-8

Fire Hydrant

Purpose: Uses buttocks and hip.
Starting Position: On all fours.
Movement: Keeping leg bent, lift one knee to the side as shown.
Goal: Beginners 25, Advanced 50.
(*fig. D-8*)

Floor Leg Crossovers

Purpose: Uses buttocks, hips and lower back as well as lower abdomen.

Starting Position: Hold bench as shown, keeping shoulders on floor, knees locked and legs as straight as possible.

Movement: Move both legs together side to side.

Goal: Beginners 10, Advanced 25.

(*fig. D-9*)

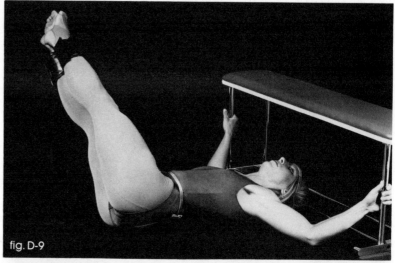
fig. D-9

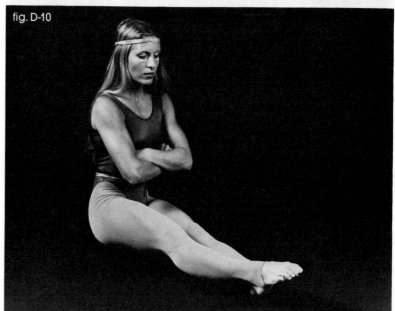
fig. D-10

Floor Walking

Sit with back straight and arms crossed. Move one cheek up and forward, proceeding across the floor. Move forward and backwards—a great pastime for when you're watching TV..

Goal: Beginners 50 steps, Advanced 100 steps.

(*figs. D-10 and 11*)

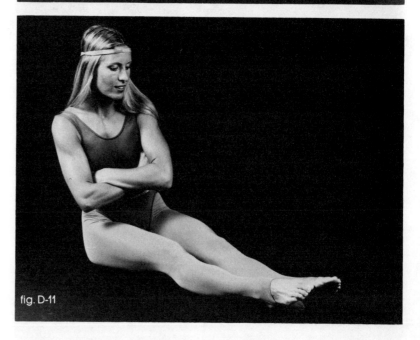
fig. D-11

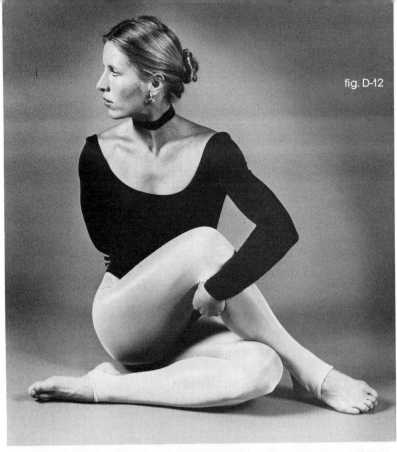

fig. D-12

The Pretzel

To reach perfection in this stretch, you must try to make your hands meet.
(*fig. D-12*)

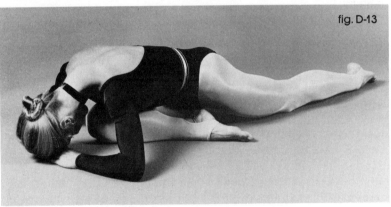

fig. D-13

The Arrow

Touch your nose to your knee.
(*fig. D-13*)

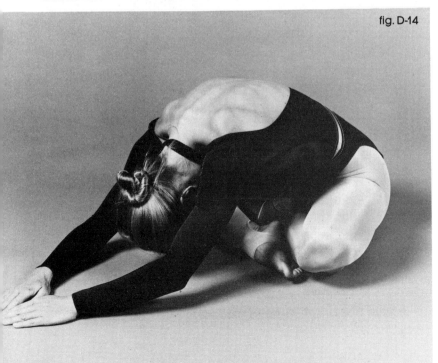

fig. D-14

Seated Bowing

One foot in front of the other, alternate feet.

Hold the above stretches for a slow 20 counts.
(*fig. D-14*)

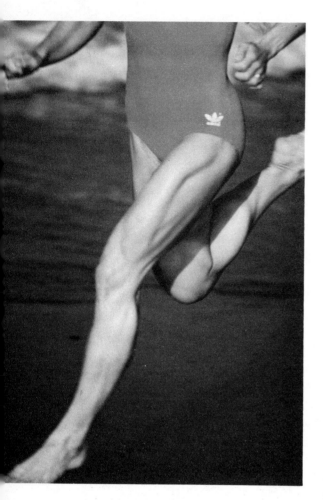

LEGS

The famous ad campaign says it all: "Nothin' beats a great pair of legs." They're right—nothing does. Your legs account for more than *half* your body structure. The femur bones are also the largest bones of the body, and attached to them are the largest muscles.

Men and women all over the world have stopped me to ask the inevitable question, "Where did you get those *legs?*" And when *Sports Illustrated* gave me the title "The Greatest Legs to Ever Stride the Earth," telegrams and letters poured in from all over the world asking the same question.

Well, they didn't just come in the mail one day. My legs used to be skinny. And once they were just plain old *fat* legs. But from each sport I've been in, from field hockey, speed skating and cycling to sprinting, modern dance and marathon running, and from each and every injury an athlete who competes as I do is almost destined to get, I've gleaned the secrets and supermethods of the Olympic athletes and star performers from all over the globe.

You can develop your legs into great legs with these methods. I've used them, and they've certainly worked for me.

What? No gym exercises in the Introduction! Are you surprised? Don't be. If someone came up with an idea that built biceps better and faster than lifting weights, people would be running outside the gyms in droves to do it. Of course, I'm not saying that the gym isn't great— it is—but it's not *the* best way and it's not even the *only* way.

When I see people doing the same old routines in the gym, I often think: How can they possibly expect to develop their legs (to be like mine) with such limited movements and repetitions?

For instance, in the course of a thirty-mile run, if you count each step as a rep, then that is thousands of reps that I do during that time. That's a lot of reps. How can you possibly stand in a gym and do one exercise that many times?

However, most marathon runners have exceptionally skinny legs, so running fifteen to thirty miles a day is certainly no guarantee of leg development.

So why did I develop and others don't? It's no big secret, but at some point you have to run *fast.* Naturally, you have to build up to it, but if you're going to run, I've always maintained that at some point you're going to have to try harder and run faster. Sprinters traditionally have more complete leg development than their distance counterparts.

If it's swimming, cycling on a stationary bicycle, or cross-country skiing or even roller skating, the same advice goes—after a two-week to four-week initial "just getting used to it" phase, try some twenty-second to thirty-second sprints where you kick harder and pump faster with your legs. This builds up your muscles' anaerobic capacity —the ability to work without oxygen—and working on this aspect of your conditioning will help give your legs shape. Start out slowly, accelerate to about 70 percent of your speed, then gradually decelerate. Try this five or eight times at the beginning. Listening to your body's reactions, include this kind of thing in your workouts at least twice a week. After several weeks, try accelerating a little more until you've upped your percentage of speed.

It's fun to go for it once in a while like this. Imagine you're overtaking your arch-rival on the home stretch and enjoy your victory!

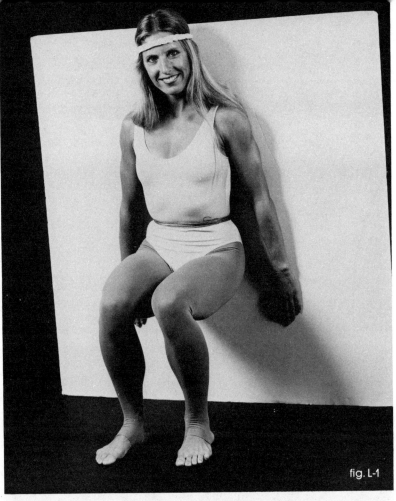

fig. L-1

Wall Sit

Purpose: Uses quadriceps.
Starting Position: Feet shoulder width apart, toes pointed straight ahead, feet roughly 18″–24″ from the wall (depending on your height).
Movement: Lower yourself into a sitting position, back, knees and feet forming perpendicular (90°) angles as if you were sitting on an invisible chair. Stay there as long as possible, timing the effort. Try to increase time with each session.
Goal: Beginners 1 minute, Advanced 5 minutes.
(*fig. L-1*)

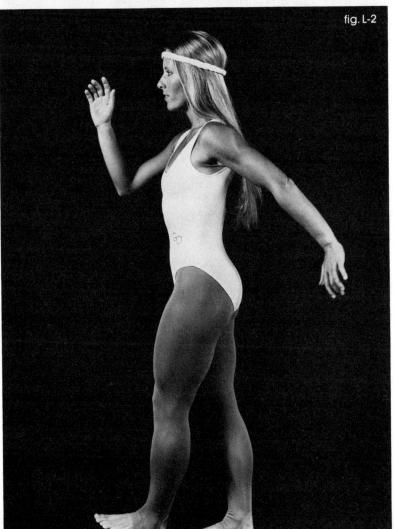

fig. L-2

Toes-up Walking

Purpose: Uses the anterior tibialis (shin).
Starting Position: Stand on heels, toes up as far as possible, with straight posture.
Movement: Take small steps. Try to increase number of steps each session.
Goal: Beginners: 50 steps, Advanced: 200 steps.
(*fig. L-2*)

Ankle Circles

Purpose: Uses shin and ankle muscles.
Starting Position: Seated with legs wide apart on the floor, flex the leg so that the heels of your feet raise up off the floor.
Movement: Make largest circles possible with your feet in both directions.
Goal: Beginners: 1 set of 30 circles in each direction, Advanced: 3 sets of 50 circles in each direction.
(*figs. L-3 and 4*)

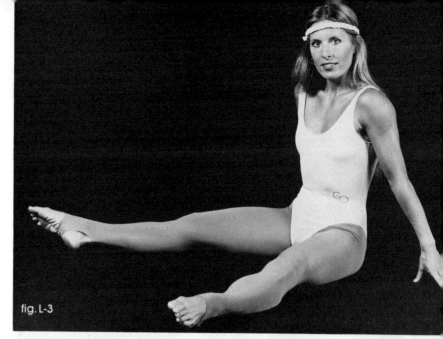

fig. L-3

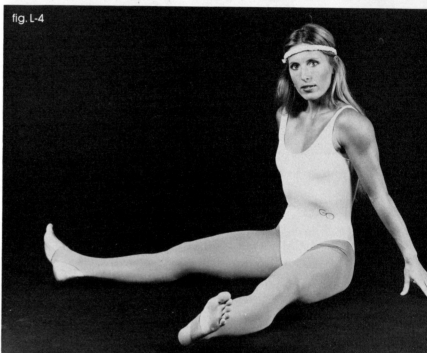

fig. L-4

Walking Lunges

Purpose: Uses groin and quadriceps.
Starting Position: Squatting, with one leg far in front of the other.
Movement: Transfer weight to front leg, then lift back leg off the ground. Straighten front leg, while leaning forward. When erect, place back leg in front, lower your body to the start position and repeat.
Goal: Beginners: 10 giant steps, Advanced: 3 sets of 20 giant steps.
(*fig. L-5*)

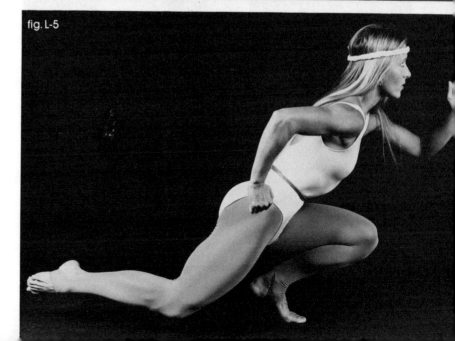

fig. L-5

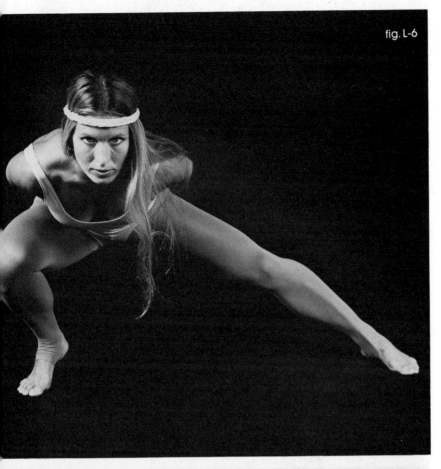

fig. L-6

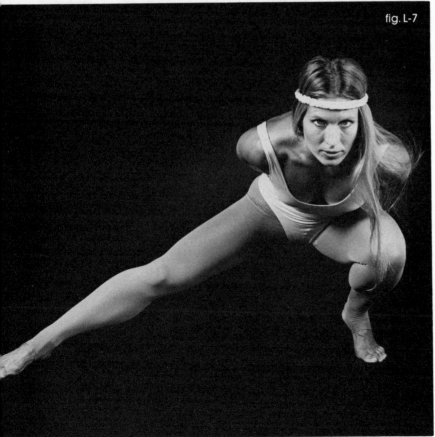

fig. L-7

Stationary Speed Skating

Purpose: Uses quadriceps, groin and buttocks.

Starting Position: Stand bent at waist as shown, with legs far apart and hands behind back.

Movement: Move body from side to side as shown, being sure to keep the body at the low height of the start position.

Goal: Beginners: (one left and one right motion equals one) 10, Advanced: 3 sets of 20. (*figs. L-6 and 7*)

Scissors with Ankle Weights

Purpose: Uses groin and lower hip.
Starting Position: Lie on floor face up as shown, with legs together and raised up.
Movement: Open legs as wide as possible. Return to starting position and repeat.
Goal: Beginners: 20 reps, Advanced: 100 reps.
(*figs. L-8 and 9*)

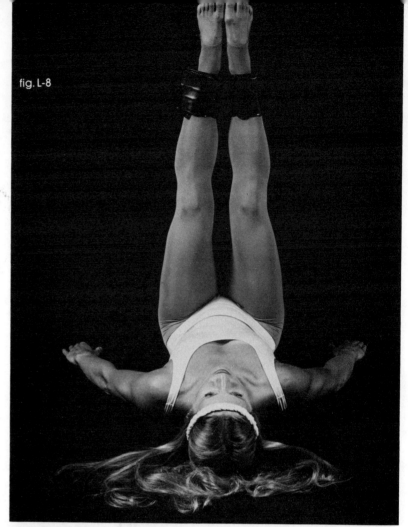

fig. L-8

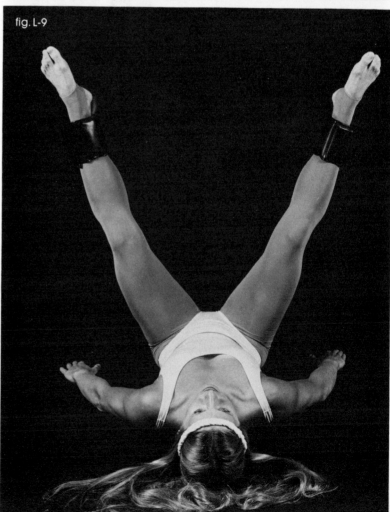

fig. L-9

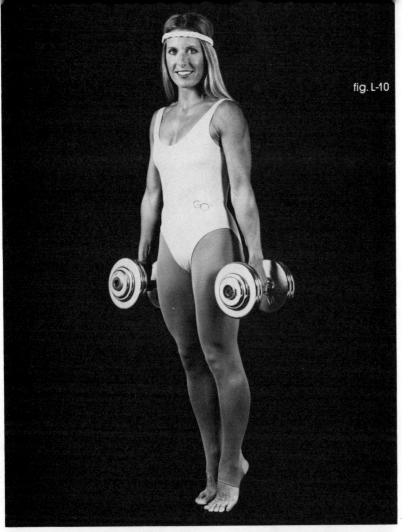

fig. L-10

Calf Raises

Purpose: Uses calves and shins. Toes pointed in uses outer calves; toes pointed out uses inner calves.

Starting Position: Feet slightly apart, toes pointed straight ahead. Grasp a dumbbell in each hand. The weight of the dumbbell can be quite heavy, as you will not be using your arms to lift it.

Movement: Raise the body weight up on your toes. Lower slowly and repeat.

Goal: Beginners: 10 reps, Advanced: 3 sets of 20 reps.

(*fig. L-10*)

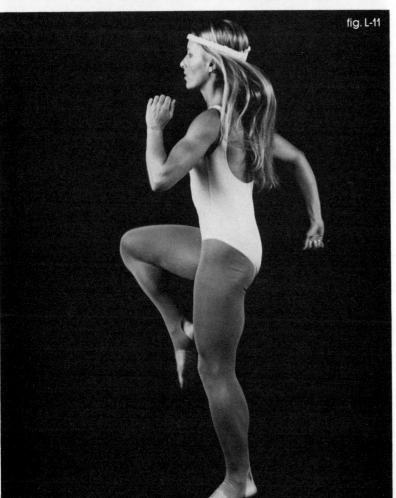

fig. L-11

High Knee Sprint

Keep back straight, pump your arms, and of course raise your knees as high as possible. Take small steps.

Goal: Beginners: 10 steps, Advanced: 25 steps.

(*fig. L-11*)

Kangaroo Jumps

Keep your knees together and try for as much height as possible.
Goal: Beginners: 10 steps, Advanced: 25 steps.
(*fig. L-12*)

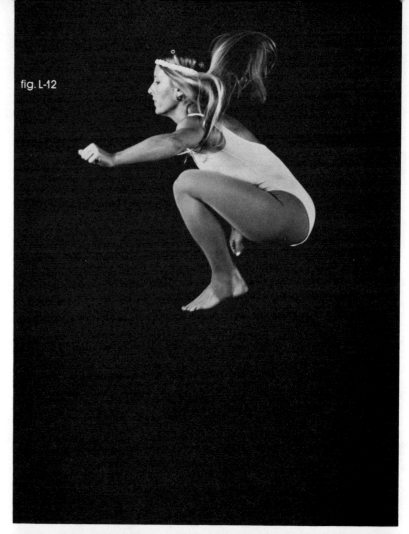

fig. L-12

Hopping

Use a driving, overemphasized arm action. Hop on one leg for the desired number of times, then alternate legs.
Goal: Beginners: 10 steps, Advanced: 25 steps.
(*fig. L-13*)

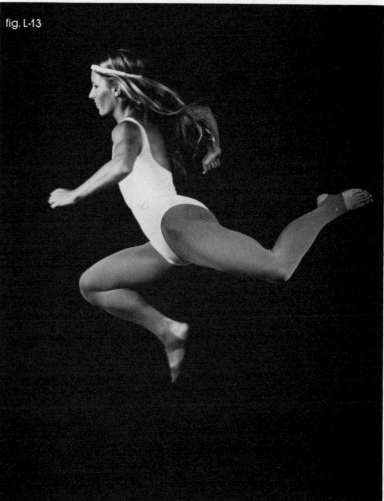

fig. L-13

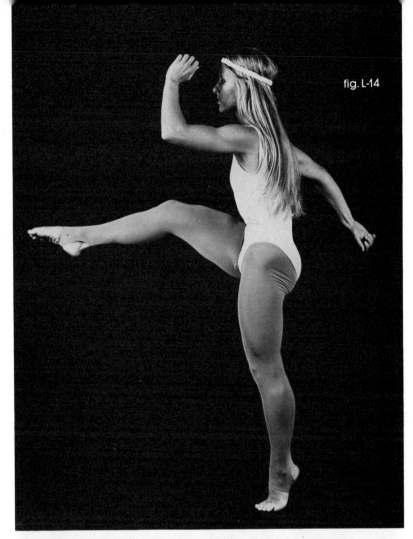

fig. L-14

Skipping March

Knee to chest, moving slowly, arms and upper body relaxed. It's the same way you skipped as a child, only extend the leg in the air before putting it down.
Goal: Beginners: 10 steps, Advanced: 25 steps.
(*fig. L-14*)

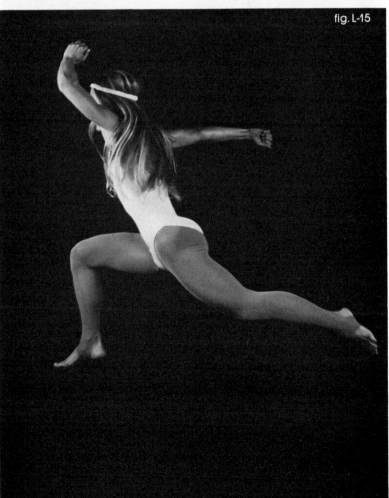

fig. L-15

Bounding

Think of running in slow motion, trying to go up as high as you can on each step.
Goal: Beginners: 10 steps, Advanced: 25 steps.
(*fig. L-15*)

LEG STRETCHING

Hold each stretch for a 50 count.

Reverse Toe Touch

(*figs. L-16 and 17*)

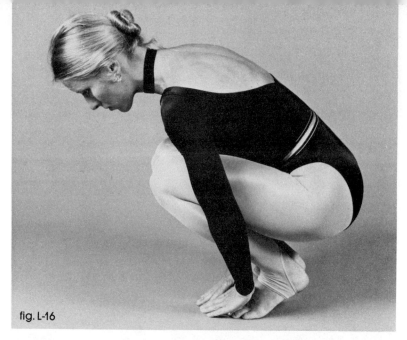

fig. L-16

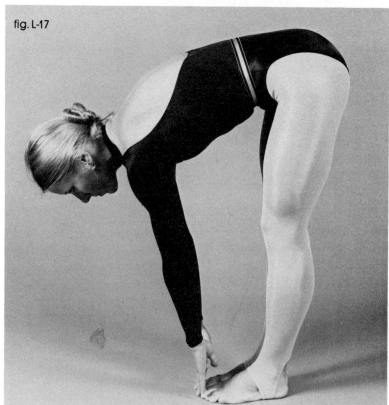

fig. L-17

Parallel Knee Hurdler's Stretch

Go just as far as is comfortable for you—don't force it.
(*fig. L-18*)

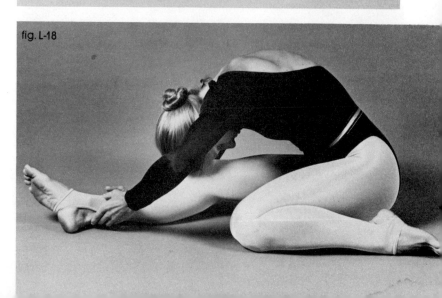

fig. L-18

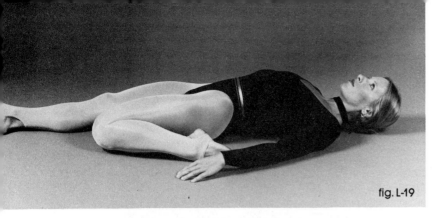

fig. L-19

Thigh Stretch

Simply lie back slowly after you have done the Parallel Hurdler's Stretch.
(*fig. L-19*)

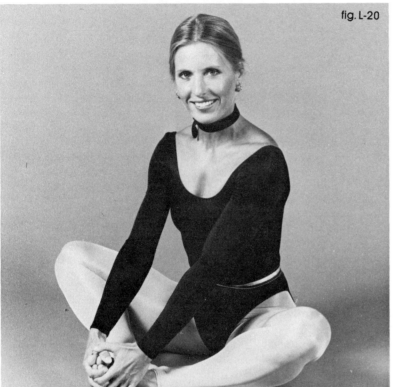

fig. L-20

Frog Sit

Soles together. The object is to bring the heels close to the body.
(*fig. L-20*)

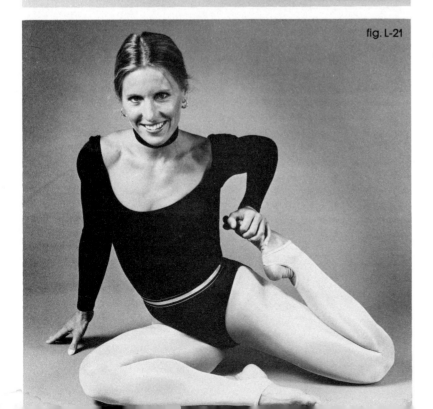

fig. L-21

Psoas Stretch

(*fig. L-21*)

Calf Stretch

With the back leg straight, put heel to floor.
Then keeping heel on the floor, bend your
knee.
(*fig. L-22*)

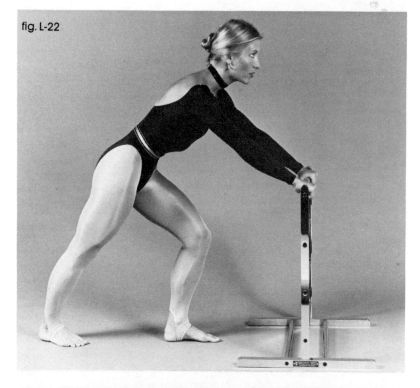

fig. L-22

Dancer's Stretch

You must press your leg down while leaning
slightly forward.
(*fig. L-23*)

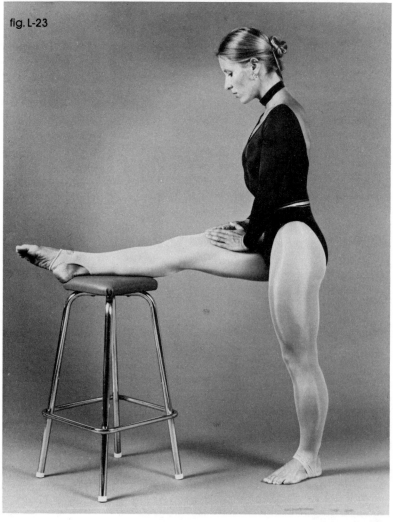

fig. L-23

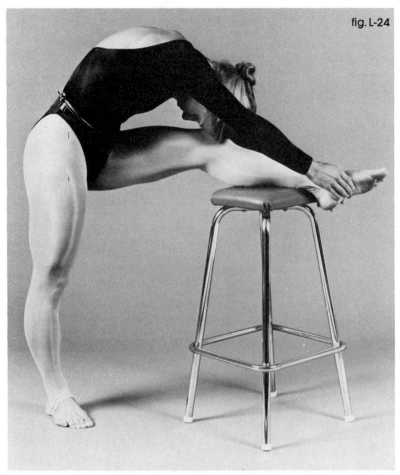

fig. L-24

Hamstring Stretch with a Stool

(*fig. L-24*)

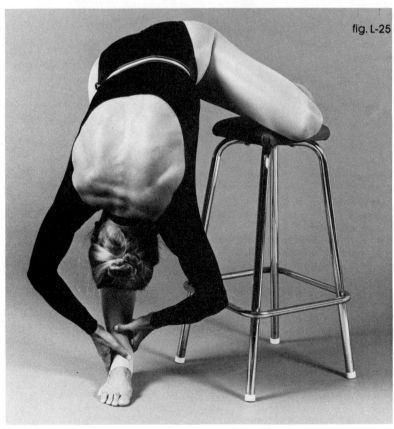

fig. L-25

Knee to Shin Straight-Leg Stretch

(*fig. L-25*)

Salute to the Sun

(*fig. L-26*)

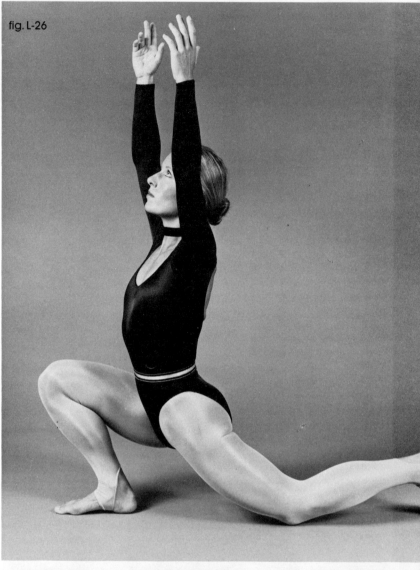

fig. L-26

Toe Crunches

Flex each foot as far as possible in the up and down position.
(*fig. F-1*)

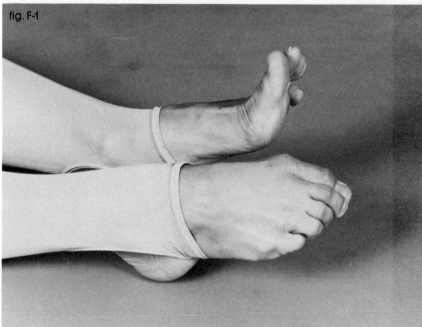

fig. F-1

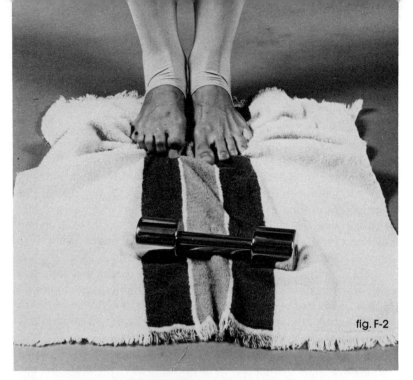

fig. F-2

Towel Toe Work

While seated in a chair, gather towel with toes.
(*fig. F-2*)

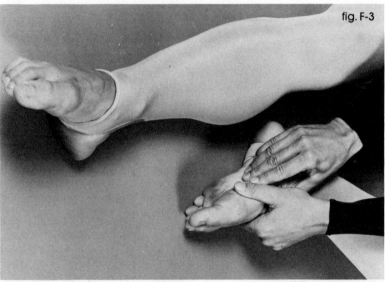

fig. F-3

Foot Massage

It is not only very gratifying for your feet, but it also helps to prevent injuries.
(*fig. F-3*)

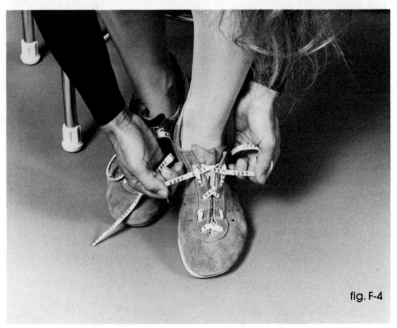

fig. F-4

How to Tie Your Shoelaces

This style of lacing your shoes allows a better fit—enabling you to "custom fit" the shoe. It can be tight or loose over the toebox and arch as desired.
(*fig. F-4*)

ARMS AND SHOULDERS

Now *these* are your show business muscles. Ask any kid to "make a muscle" and you'll always get a bicep flex.

The biceps, triceps, forearms and deltoids are the muscles that are most often in the spotlight. Weakness here in any one of these muscles could impair even the simplest of everyday tasks such as brushing your teeth. Flexion and extension of the elbow is the main function of the biceps and triceps. The forearms are of prime importance in the racquet sports, where hand grip is imperative.

Shoulders are extremely important to runners and swimmers. Even walking employs the deltoids. Naturally, mountain climbers, pole vaulters, gymnasts and skiers use their deltoids daily. I've noticed that speed skating and rowing causes tiredness in my shoulders, but if you'd really like a different shoulder workout, allow me to suggest conducting a symphony orchestra for several hours!

Strong sinewy arms are an attribute to any woman or man, and it's interesting to note that in calculating the body's percentage of fat, technicians always use the calipers under your tricep. The saying is that if you can "pinch an inch" there, you are overfed and underexercised.

For runners, developing your deltoids can help not only your stride length but also your speed. Similarly in swimming, stroke power and body speed rely on the shoulders.

And if you've ever wanted to contribute to the illusion of a small, tapering waist, building your shoulders is a sure bet. So nose to the grindstone, and shoulder to the wheel—this section is for you.

BICEPS

Bicep Curl

Purpose: Uses biceps.
Starting Position: Stand facing mirror with feet apart, dumbbells at sides. You may also be seated.
Movement: Curl the dumbbell toward your shoulder. Lower and repeat with other arm.
Goal: Beginners and Advanced: Use a weight with which you can do 3 sets of 10 repetitions. Increase the weight as 3 sets become comfortable.
(*fig. A-1*)

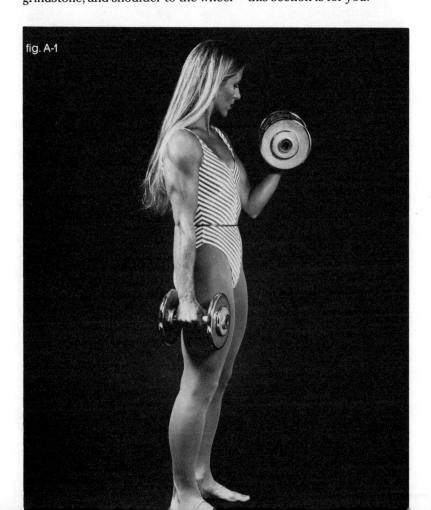

fig. A-1

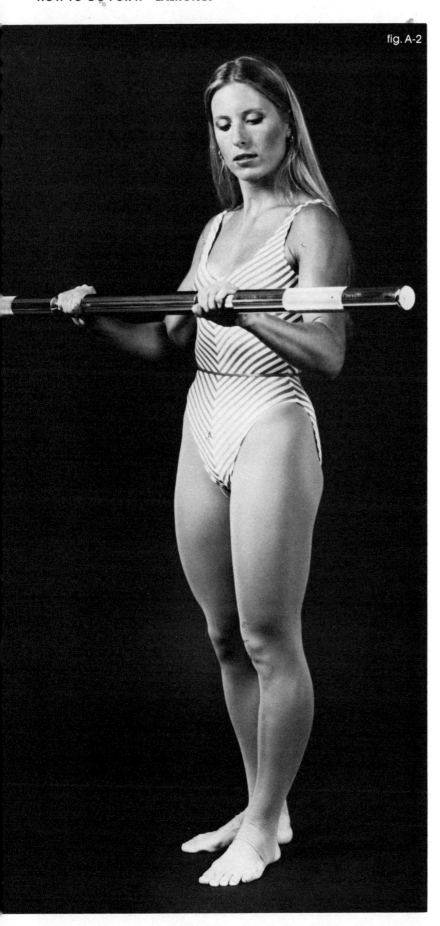

fig. A-2

Reverse Curl with Bar

Purpose: Uses biceps and brachialis muscle, as well as forearms.

Starting Position: Stand facing mirror with feet apart. Grip bar, palms away, bar resting on upper thighs.

Movement: Bring bar up toward shoulders, using elbows as a pivotal point. Keep arms close to the body. Lower bar and repeat.

Goal: See Bicep Curl, page 52.

(*fig. A-2*)

Concentration Curl

Purpose: Isolates the biceps and uses it deep into the muscle.

Starting Position: Sit on the edge of a bench or chair. Grasp dumbbell in one hand and lean forward. Immobilize the elbow of that arm by pressing it into the inside of the thigh as shown.

Movement: Curl the dumbbell to the shoulder, pausing at the top, then lowering slowly. Repeat for desired number of slowly. Repeat for desired number of repetitions, then switch to other arm.

Goal: See Bicep Curl, page 52.

(*figs. A-3 and 4*)

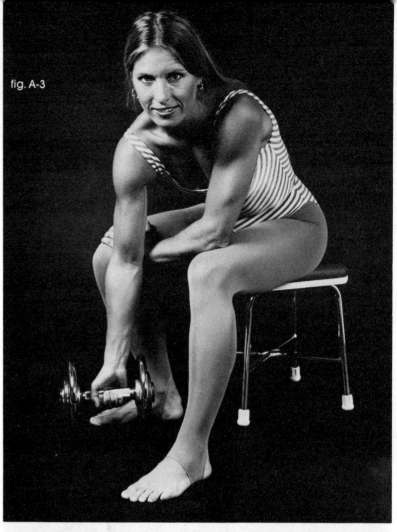

fig. A-3

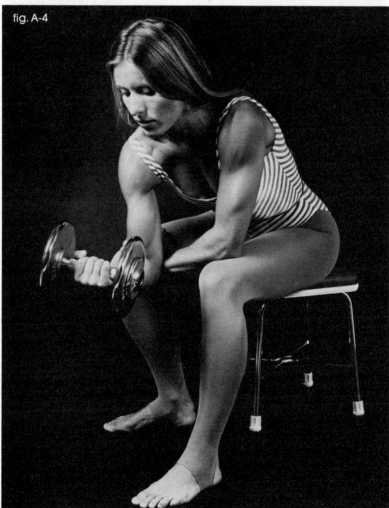

fig. A-4

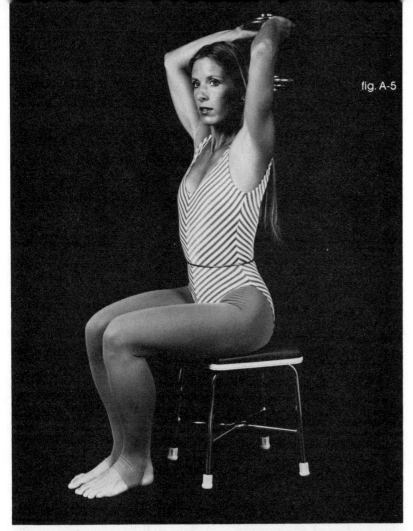

fig. A-5

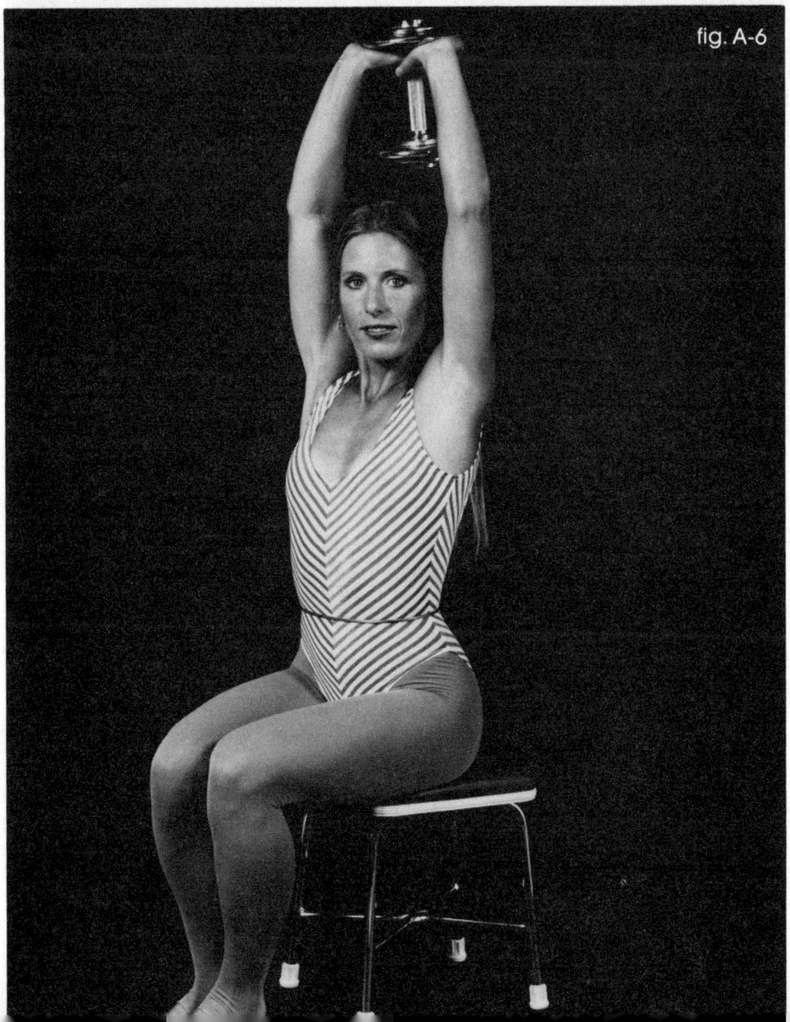

TRICEPS

Seated Dumbbell Tricep Curl

Purpose: Uses triceps.
Starting Position: Sit on bench or chair as shown, one hand grasping dumbbell, elbow bent and arm close to head. Other hand is helping to keep the elbow in position.
Movement: Keeping arm close to head, raise the dumbbell. Think of the elbow as a pivot— only the hand and dumbbell move. Your palm will open as the weight reaches the top position.
Goal: See Bicep Curl, page 52.
(*figs. A-5 and 6*)

fig. A-6

Tricep Push-ups

Purpose: Uses triceps.
Starting Position: Lie face down on the
floor with your weight supported by the hands
and toes. Fingers will point toward each
opposite hand.
Movement: Extend arms, keeping body rigid
and straight. Lower and repeat.
Goal: Beginners: Your goal is to reach 10.
Start with whatever you can do keeping good
form—1 perfect rep is good. Advanced: 3 sets
of 10.
(*figs. A-9 and 10*)

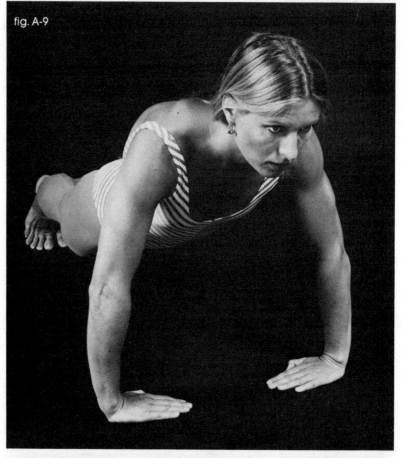

fig. A-9

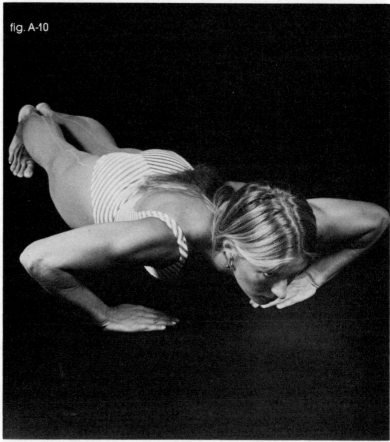

fig. A-10

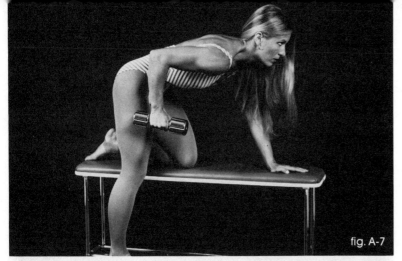

fig. A-7

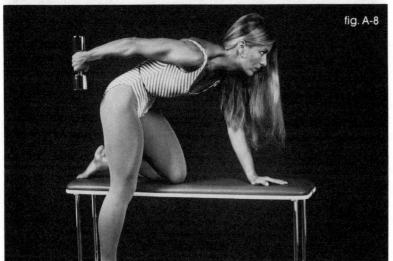

fig. A-8

Back Arm Curl

Purpose: Uses triceps.
Starting Position: Lean one hand and one leg on bench as shown, grasping the dumbbell in your other hand.
Movement: As in the seated tricep curl, your elbow is only a pivot and does not move. Extend the dumbbell backward. Return to start position, keeping arm close to body. Repeat.
Goal: See Bicep Curl, page 52.
(*figs. A-7 and 8*)

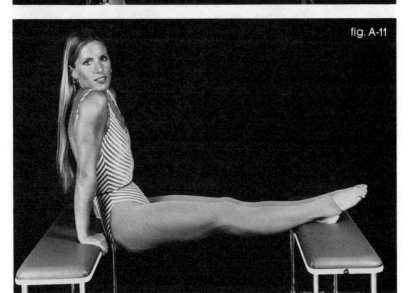

fig. A-11

Tricep Dips on a Bench

Purpose: Uses triceps and shoulders.
Starting Position: Position yourself between two chairs or benches as shown, with heels resting on one bench.
Movement: Extend arms, but do not lock elbows at the top position. Lower yourself and repeat.
Goal: Beginner: 10 reps, Advanced: 3 sets of 10 reps.
(*figs. A-11 and 12*)

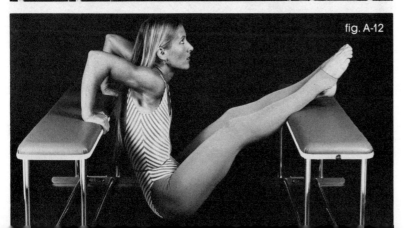

fig. A-12

DELTOIDS

Seated or Standing Dumbbell Presses

Purpose: Uses the front and outer deltoids.
Starting Position: Grasp dumbbell in each hand and hold at shoulder level.
Movement: Press the dumbbells overhead and lower slowly back to the start position. Repeat.
Goal: Beginners and Advanced: Use a weight with which you can do 3 sets of 10 repetitions. Increase the weight as 3 sets become comfortable.
(*figs. A-13 and 14*)

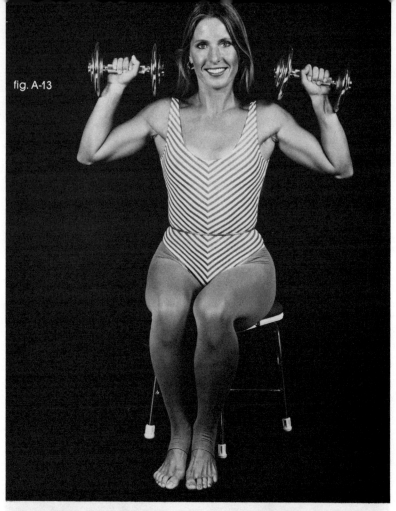

fig. A-13

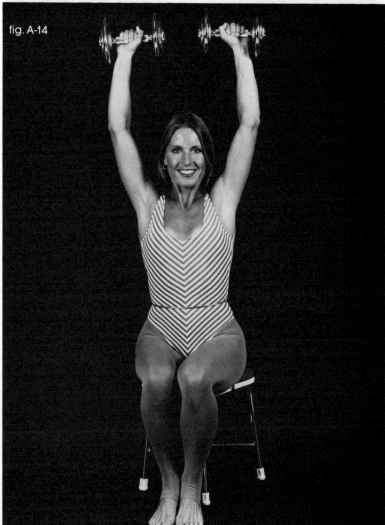

fig. A-14

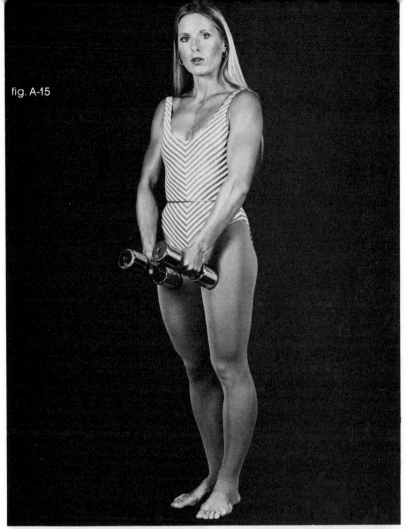

fig. A-15

Flys

Purpose: Uses front and outer deltoids.
Starting Position: Stand facing mirror with feet slightly apart, a dumbbell in each hand and resting on upper thighs.
Movement: Inhale while sweeping arms up to shoulder height. Keep arms fairly straight but think of your elbows as leading the arms up. Pause at the top and straighten your arms completely while in that position. Return arms slowly to start position and repeat.
Goal: See Dumbbell Presses, p. 58.
(*figs. A-15 and 16*)

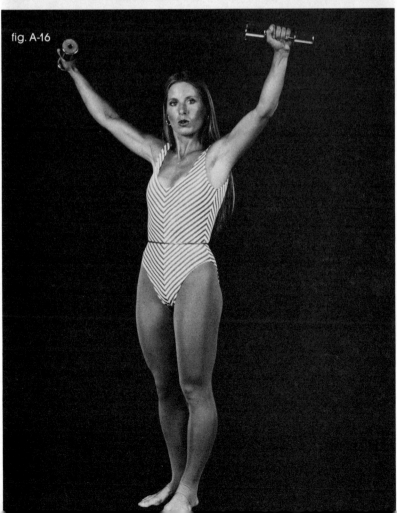

fig. A-16

Robot Flys

Purpose: Uses the front deltoids.
Starting Position: Stand facing the mirror with feet slightly apart, a dumbbell in each hand and resting on the upper thighs.
Movement: Bring the dumbbell up to shoulder height, keeping arm straight. Lower and repeat with other arm.
Goal: See Dumbbell Presses, p. 58.
(*figs. A-17 and 18*)

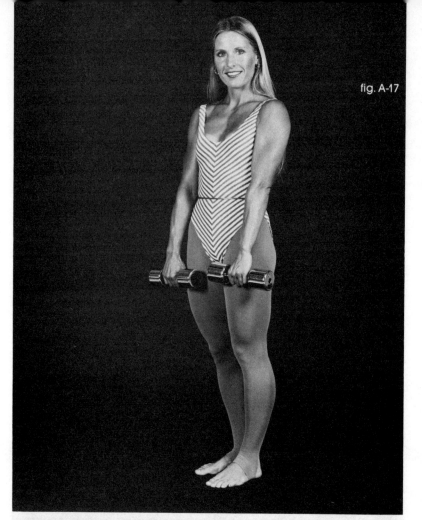

fig. A-17

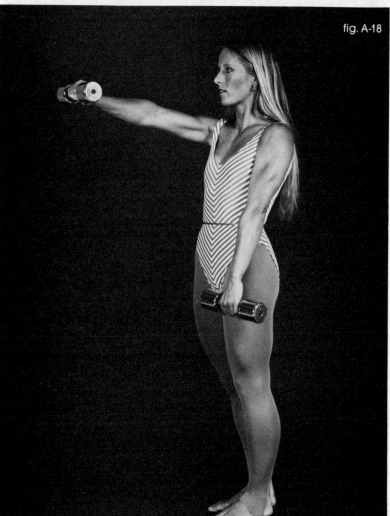

fig. A-18

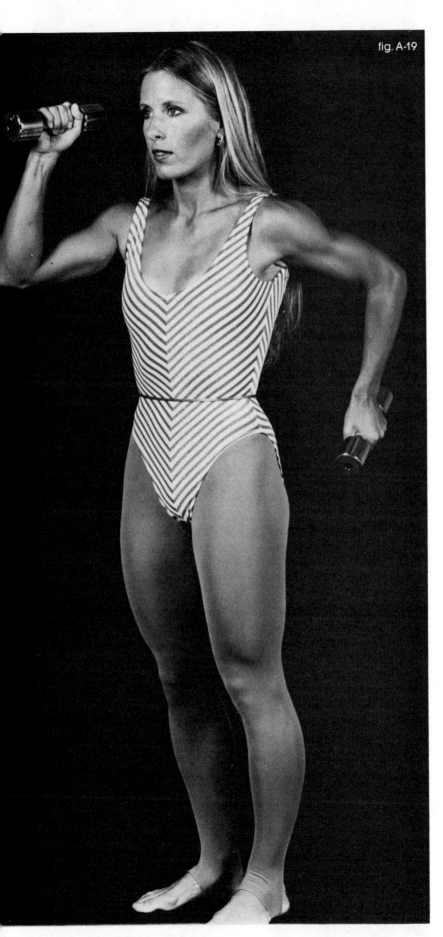

fig. A-19

Running Arms

Purpose: Uses back part of deltoids and triceps. Helps correct running form and aids in developing speed.

Starting Position: Stand facing mirror with feet slightly apart. Grasp a dumbbell in each hand, arms at a perpendicular (90°) angle.

Movement: Using the shoulder as a pivotal point, swing arms back and forward in a rapid running motion. Choose a light weight and repeat many times. You may want to do this for a timed set rather than for a specific number of repetitions—for example, 2 minutes with good form.

Goal: Beginners: 1 minute, Advanced: 3 minutes.

(*fig. A-19*)

FOREARMS

All exercises using a dumbbell or barbell or
bar require the use of the forearms in order to
grip the weight. The following exercises are
specifically for the forearm.

Seated Dumbbell Wrist Curl

Purpose: Uses forearms.
Starting Position: Sit on edge of chair or
bench as shown, with feet elevated (a box or
several telephone directories will do). Grasp
dumbbells, palms up, and keep back of the
forearms supported by your thighs.
Movement: Curl the dumbbell up as far as
possible, keeping the arms immobile and
using the wrist as a pivot. Then slowly and
carefully allow the dumbbell to roll back with
your hand until only the fingers are
supporting it. Repeat, pausing at the top and
bottom position of the movement.
Goal: Beginners and Advanced: Use a weight
with which you can do 3 sets of 10 repetitions.
Increase the weight as 3 sets become
comfortable.
(*figs. A-20 and 21*)

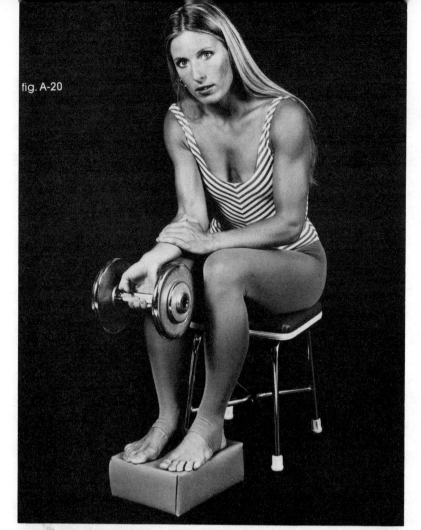

fig. A-20

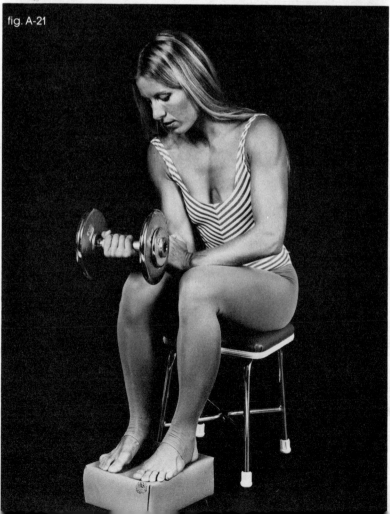

fig. A-21

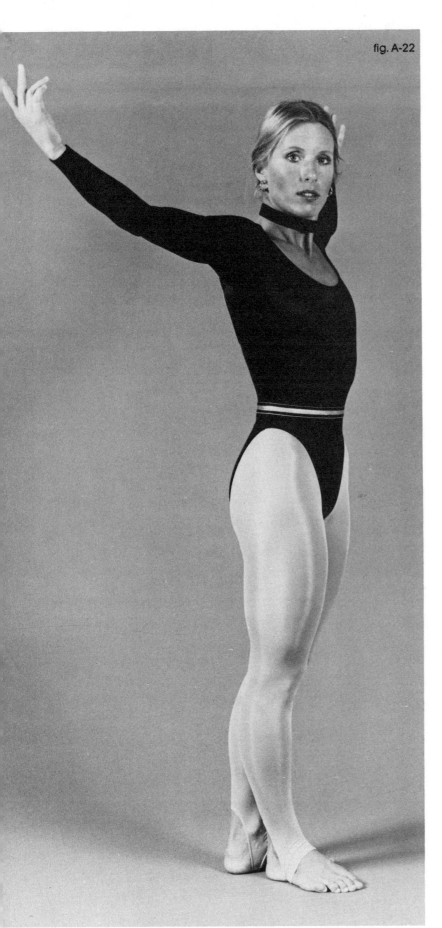

fig. A-22

ARM STRETCHES

Full Arm Circles in Each Direction

(*fig. A-22*)
Do 5 rotations in each direction.

Towel Stretch

Pull towel downwards with the bottom hand.
Hold for a 50 count. Repeat for other arm.
(*fig. A-23*)

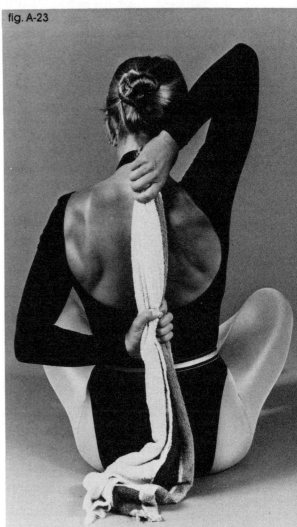

fig. A-23

CHEST

Athletes often neglect working on their chest because it's not one of the classic flashy muscles like those of the arm or leg.

But the only muscles used by the body more than the heart, which pumps continuously, are the chest muscles. Each breath you take requires the chest to expand and contract. Most people do not realize that filling the lungs with air is really caused by the muscular contraction of the pectoral and intercostal muscles, which in turn sets up a vacuum, causing air to rush in to the lungs. Any muscle that important surely deserves more respect.

In addition, women will be pleased to learn that a more voluptuous bosom and cleavage between the breasts can be achieved by developing the pectoral muscles.

In men and women, a sweep of developed pectorals adds to the effect of wide shoulders, thus enhancing the look of a narrow waist.

Dumbbell Bench Press

Purpose: Uses the outer chest.
Starting Position: While sitting on the floor or bench take a dumbbell in each hand and rest them on your lap. Lie back on the bench or floor, straightening your arms over your chest.
Movement: With the dumbbells in the air, bend your arms and lower them in a semicircular fashion, keeping your elbows wide. Return to start position and repeat.
Goal: Beginners and Advanced: Use a weight with which you can do 3 sets of 10 repetitions. Increase the weight as 3 sets become comfortable.
(*figs. C-1 and 2*)

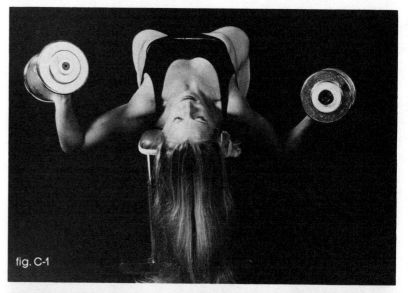
fig. C-1

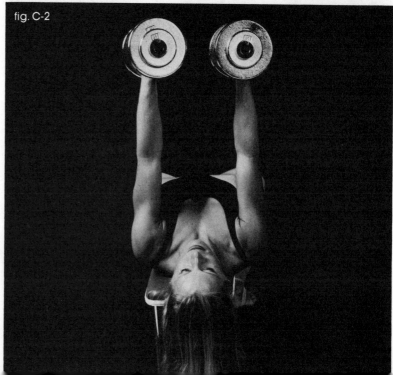
fig. C-2

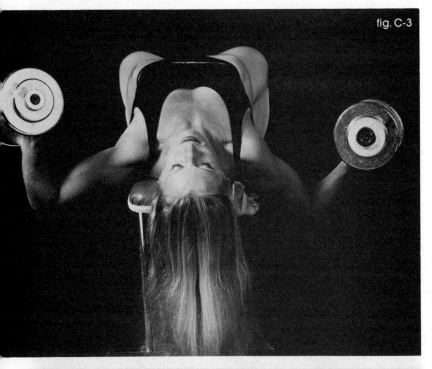

fig. C-3

Dumbbell Crossovers

Purpose: Uses the outer, inner and upper chest.
Starting Position: Same as dumbbell bench press.
Movement: With the dumbbells in the air, bend your arms and lower them in a semicircular fashion, keeping your elbows wide. Return past the starting position, crossing your arms over your chest. Repeat.
Goal: See above.
(*figs. C-3 and 4*)

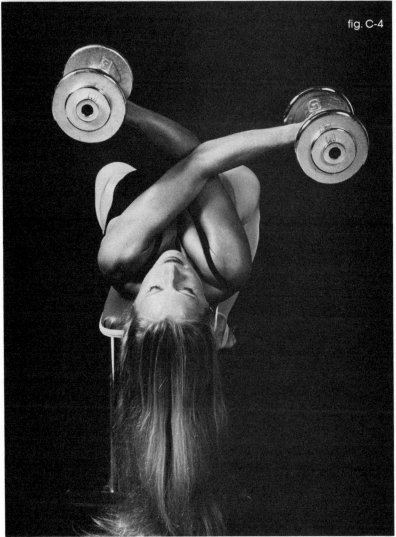

fig. C-4

Straight Dumbbell Pullover

Purpose: Uses the chest and rib cage.
Starting Position: Hold one dumbbell in a straight-arm position over the chest using both hands, palms up.
Movement: Lower the dumbbell behind your head in a semicircular movement while bending elbows. Return to start position and repeat. The hands will move naturally from a palms-up to a slight palms-together position as you lower the dumbbell.
Goal: See above.
(*figs. C-5 and 6*)

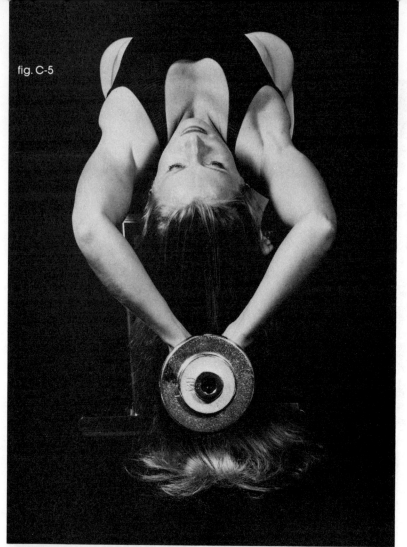

fig. C-5

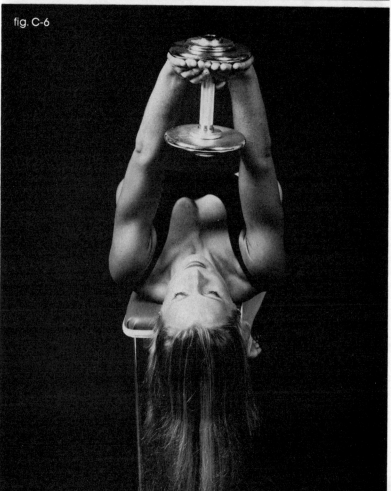

fig. C-6

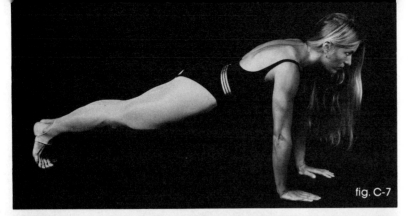

fig. C-7

Push-ups

Purpose: Uses the chest and triceps. Hands 6″ apart: inner chest and triceps. Hands 24″ apart: mid-chest and shoulders. Hands 36″ apart: outer chest, shoulders and lats (Latissimus dorsi) (back).

Starting Position: Lie face down on the floor, with your weight supported by the hands and toes.

Movement: Push the arms straight while keeping the body rigid. Lower slowly and repeat.

Goal: Beginners: Your goal is to reach 10. Start with whatever you can do keeping good form. 1 perfect push-up is good. Advanced: 3 sets of 10.

(*figs. C-7 and 8*)

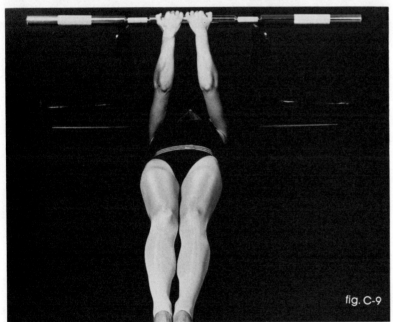

fig. C-8

Chin-ups

Purpose: Uses inner chest, biceps.

Starting Position: Close grip, palms facing in for inner chest. Wide grip, palms facing in for outer chest.

Movement: Pull your chin up to the bar, lower and repeat.

Goal: Beginners: Your goal is to reach 10. Start with whatever you can do keeping good form. 1 perfect chin is good. If you can't do 1, use a chair. Stand on chair with your chin up to the bar. Then lower yourself. As you get stronger, you won't need the chair. Advanced: 3 sets of 10.

Chin-up Variation with Chair

Starting Position: Position your chest under the bar. Grasp bar with palms facing in. Keep body straight.

Movement: Pull your chest to the bar, keeping body straight and heels touching the floor. Lower and repeat.

Goal: Beginners: 10 reps, Advanced: 3 sets of 10 reps.

(*figs. C-9 and 10*)

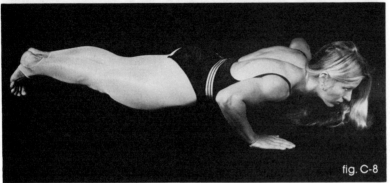

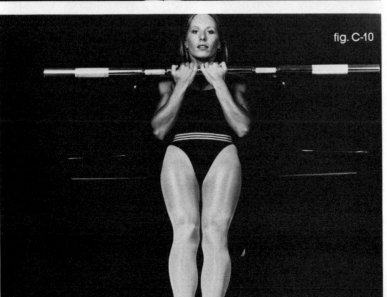

fig. C-9

fig. C-10

Towel Chest Stretch

Bring arms slowly behind your back until they touch your body. Then bring them back up over your head.
(*fig. C-11*)

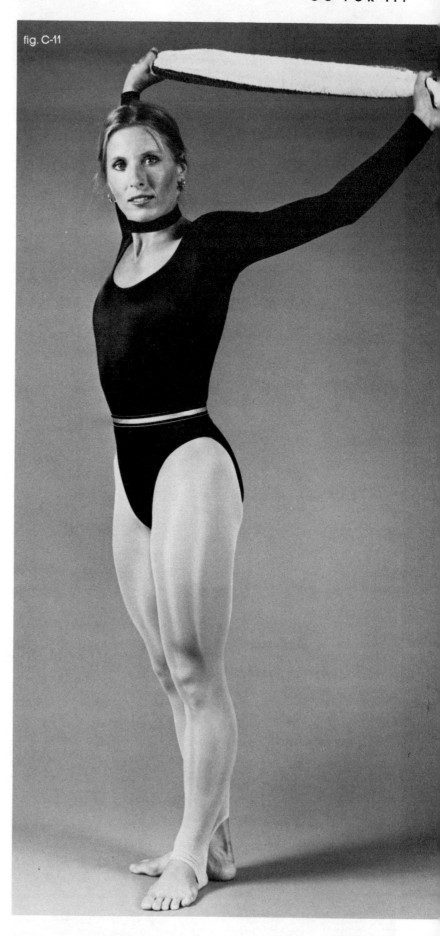

fig. C-11

THE BACK

The back, mighty and strong, is able to resist even the powerful force of the earth's gravity. Weak, it reduces us to a bent-over hunch —impairing our ability to stand erect, walk or even breathe correctly.

The back, consisting mainly of the lateral and spinal erectors, as well as the trapezius and lumbar dorsals, is the source of great power and speed in the body. Yet even though it is capable of enormous strength, if you've ever strained your back, you know just how debilitating it can be. "Oh, my aching back!" is a complaint heard all too frequently, and usually because of complete unawareness of how to strengthen it. Women also abuse their backs by wearing high-heeled shoes, which force the spine into a "swayback" position, weakening and straining the lower vertebrae of the spine.

Stability of the back prevents injuries to many different body parts, including feet, knees, neck and shoulders.

It is important to every movement of the body, and when you consider that these muscles protect our spinal columns and the central nervous system, this should be more than motivation enough to develop the area. Building your back is like an insurance policy on your spine, and you will be rewarded with the sinewy grace of a powerful back that can be yours for as long as you live.

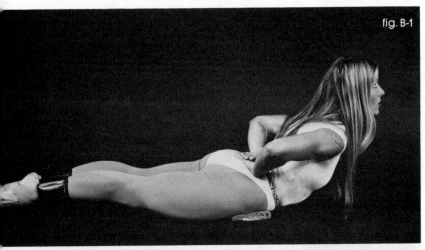

fig. B-1

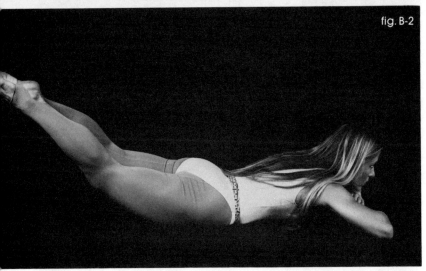

fig. B-2

Hyperextension

Purpose: Uses low back.
Starting Position: Lie face down on the floor with a rolled towel at pelvis.
Movement: Raise trunk off floor slowly. Lower and repeat.
(*figs. B-1 and 2*)

Hyperextension Variation

Movement: Raise both legs off the floor. Lower and repeat.
Goal: Beginners: 10 reps, Advanced: 3 sets of 10.

A FEW TIPS

A few tips for your back and how to get along with it and help yourself out if it bothers you.

Before the workout, try jogging on the spot for a few minutes to warm up. Make sure you wear a shirt that tucks in—it is easy to catch a draft on your back. Here are some things you should always be doing for a strong, healthy back.

Sitting—Use a hard chair and put your spine up against it—try to keep one or both knees higher than your hips. A small stool or several telephone books under your feet are more comfortable here.

Standing—Try to stand with your lower back flat.

Sleeping—Sleep on a firm mattress. Do not sleep on your stomach. If you sleep on your back, put a pillow under your knees. If you sleep on your side, keep legs bent at the knees and hips.

At Work—If you work at a desk, get up and move around whenever you get the chance, and be sure to stretch frequently. If your job requires you to lift things, bend your knees and use your legs to help you. Be certain the load is light enough for you to manage comfortably. This is not the time to be a hero. When bending over—even if it's only to open a file cabinet, or pick up a pencil—do not bend at the waist, bend at the knees.

Pull-ups

Purpose: Uses latissimus dorsi ("lats") and shoulder muscles.
Close grip: lower latissimus dorsi erecter
Medium grip: general.
Wide grip: upper latissimus dorsi.
Starting Position: Grasp bar, palms facing away.
Movement: Pull body up to the bar. Lower and repeat.
Goal: Beginners: 5 is your goal. Start with 1 perfect pull-up. If you can't do 1, use a chair and stand with neck up to the bar. Then lower yourself. Advanced: 3 sets of 5.
(*figs. B-3 and 4*)

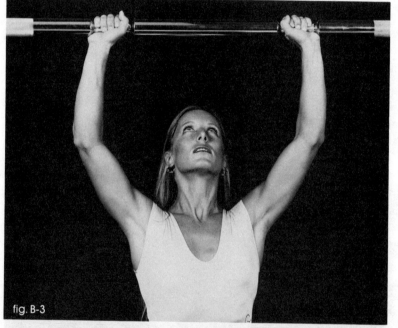

fig. B-3

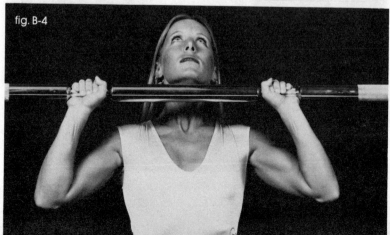

fig. B-4

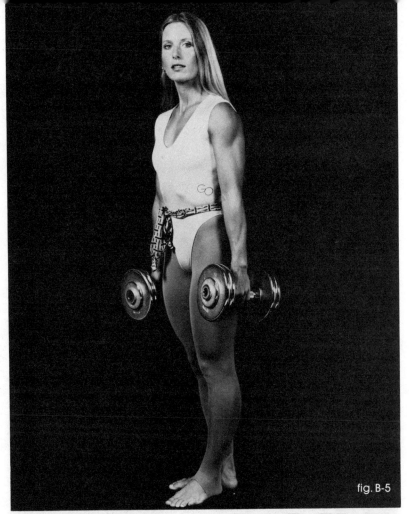

fig. B-5

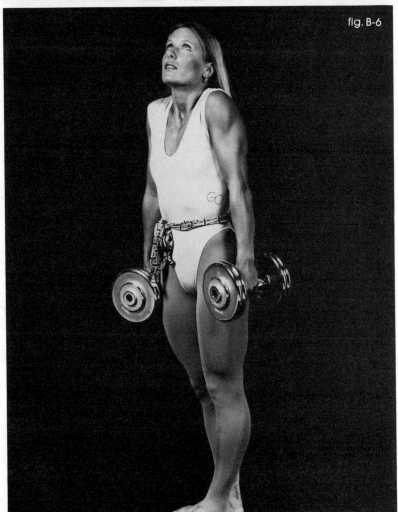

fig. B-6

Shoulder Shrugs

Purpose: Uses trapezius muscles. Relieves tension in neck.

Starting Position: Stand facing mirror, feet shoulder width apart, holding dumbbells at sides.

Movement: Move shoulders up toward ears, keeping back straight. You may also be seated for this exercise.

Goal: Advanced and Beginners: Use a weight with which you can do 3 sets of 10 repetitions. Increase the weight as 3 sets become comfortable.

(*figs. B-5 and 6*)

Bent Rowing, One Arm

Purpose: Uses upper and lower lats and shoulders.
Starting Position: One hand and one leg on bench as shown. Grasp dumbbell and turn hand to a 45° angle with other hand.
Movement: Bring the dumbbell up to the lower rib cage. Lower and repeat for required number of repetitions. Repeat with other arm.
Goal: See Shoulder Shrugs, page 71.
(*figs. B-7 and 8*)

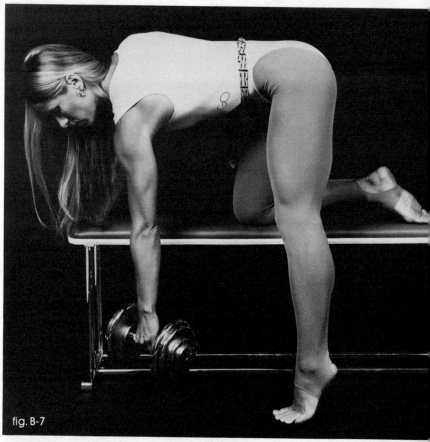

fig. B-7

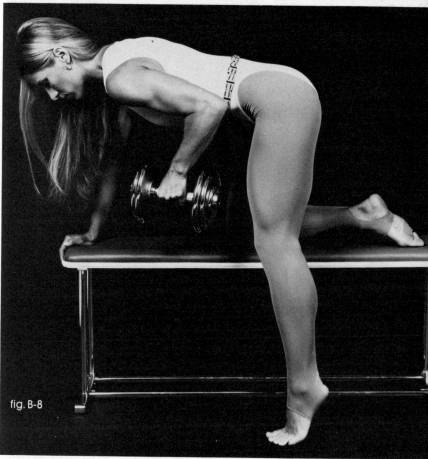

fig. B-8

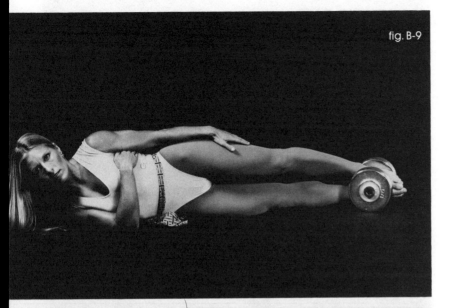

fig. B-9

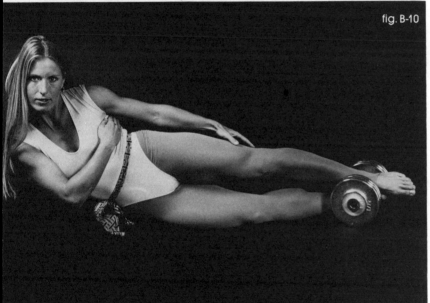

fig. B-10

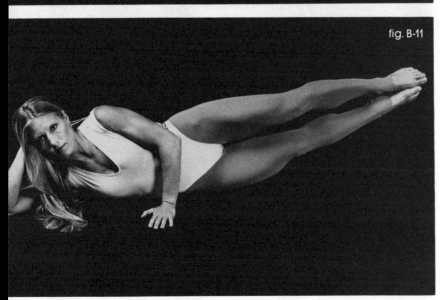

fig. B-11

Side Trunk Raises and Double Leg Raises

Purpose: Uses low back and hip muscles.

Starting Position: Lie on your side as shown, with bottom arm crossing chest, and top arm straight along the body.

Movement: (Side Trunk Raises) Raise trunk off the floor, keep the back in a line. Lower and repeat.

Movement: (Double Leg Raises) Using the same starting position, raise both legs slowly. Lower and repeat.

Goal: Beginners: 10 reps is your goal. Start with the number of repetitions you can do keeping good form on each side. Advanced: 3 sets of 10.

(figs. B-9, 10 and 11)

Standing Upright Row

Purpose: Uses upper back between shoulder blades and trapezius muscles.

Starting Position: Stand facing the mirror with feet slightly apart and dumbbells resting against upper thighs.

Movement: Keeping elbows apart and dumbbells 10″ apart, raise the dumbbells to shoulders. Keep the dumbbells close to the body. Lower and repeat.

Goal: See Shoulder Shrugs, page 71. (*figs. B-12 and 13*)

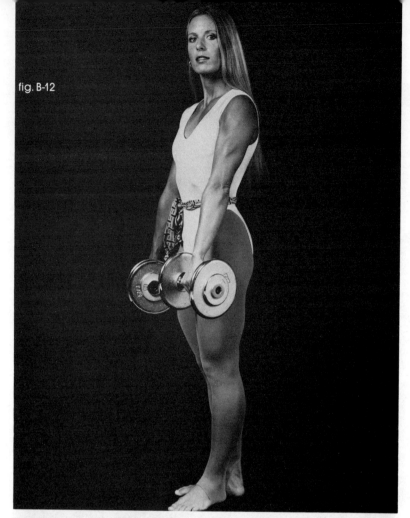

fig. B-12

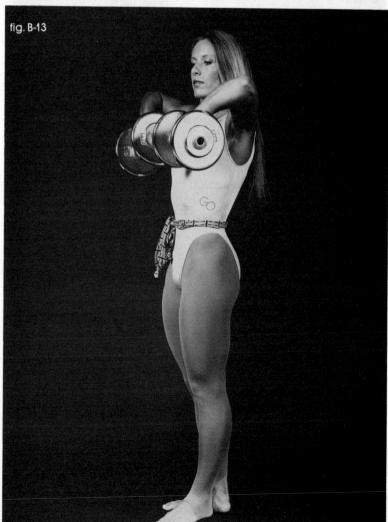

fig. B-13

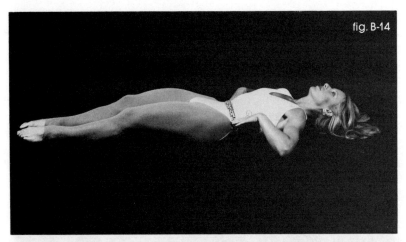

fig. B-14

Back Press

Purpose: Uses low back.
Starting Position: Lie on your back on the floor.
Movement: Press the small of your back into the floor. Hold for several seconds. Relax and repeat.
Goal: Beginners: Hold for a slow 10 count. Repeat 5 times. Advanced: Hold for a slow 20 count. Repeat 5 times.
(*fig. B-14*)

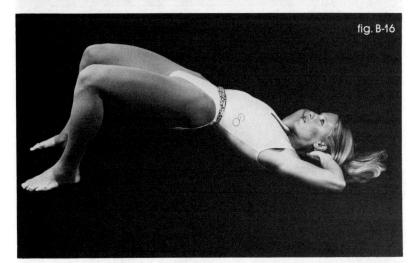

fig. B-15

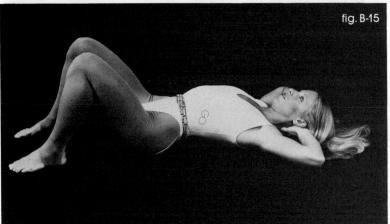

fig. B-16

Pelvic Lift

Feet shoulder width apart—hold the top position for a few seconds.
(*figs. B-15 and 16*)

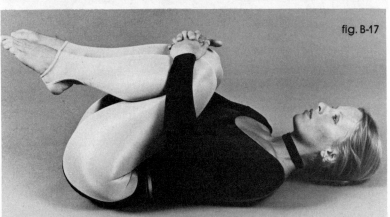

fig. B-17

Knee to Chest Stretch

Hold for a 50 count.
(*fig. B-17*)

MORE BACK STRETCHING

Heels Over Head

Keep knees bent. Hold for a 50 count.
(*fig. B-18*)

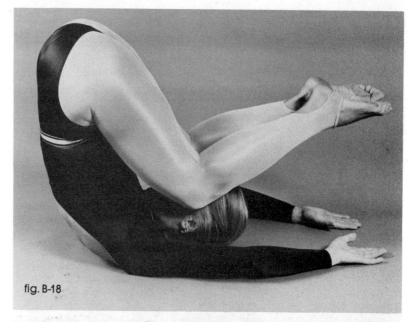

fig. B-18

The Umbrella

Hands shoulder width apart. As you improve,
bring your hands closer to your feet. Hold for
a 50 count.
(*fig. B-19*)

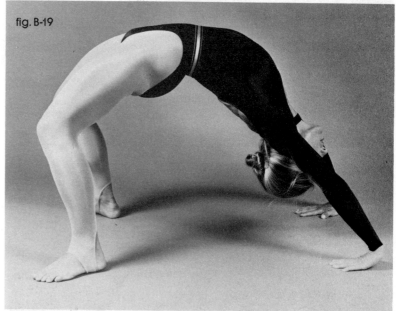

fig. B-19

Child Sleep Position

A very relaxing position, especially at the end
of the day. Hold for a 50 count.
(*fig. B-20*)

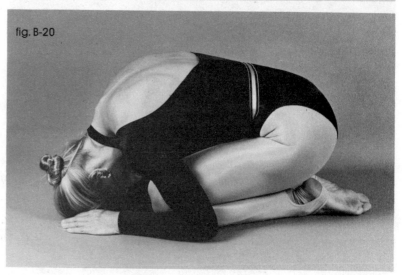

fig. B-20

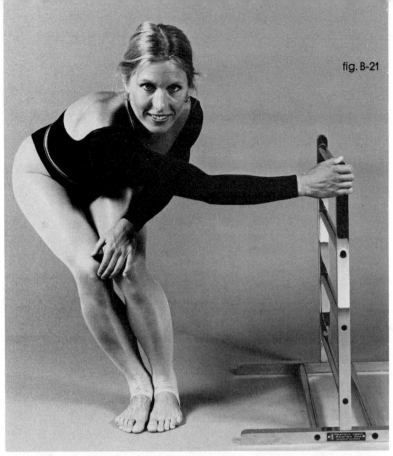

fig. B-21

Side Lat Muscle Stretch

Gently pull with your straight arm. Hold for a 50 count.
(*fig. B-21*)

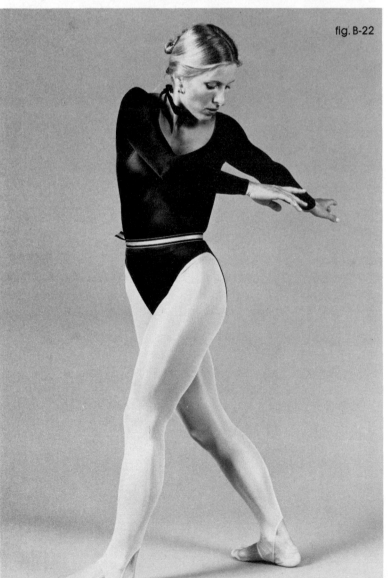

fig. B-22

Twist and Look

Feet at shoulder width. Swing arms around with momentum, twisting your trunk and looking at that back heel. Repeat 5–10 times.
(*fig. B-22*)

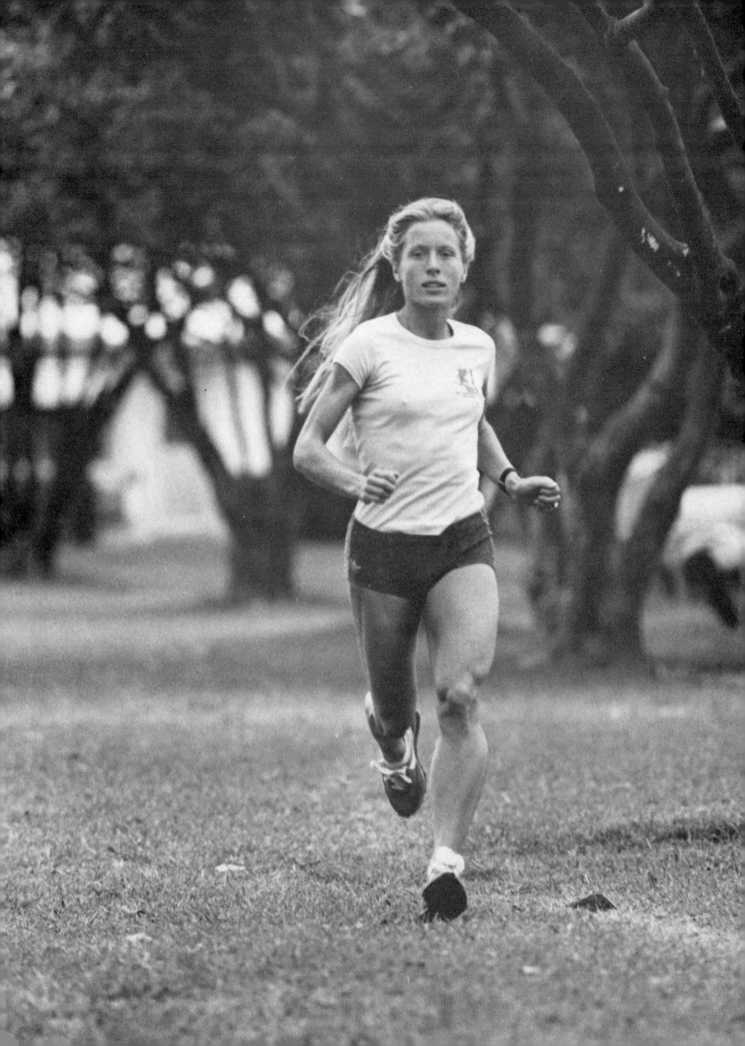

3
AEROBICS AND THE HEART

THE HEART

Poets, songwriters and incurable romantics of all ages have always believed that the heart is what rules us. Now, exercise psychologists and scientists are confirming the fact.

While lifting weights will give your skeletal muscles the opportunity to get stronger, the effect upon the heart is not enough for necessary cardiovascular fitness. You must also engage in some kind of activity that will enable your heart to beat faster and become stronger (aerobic activity).

HOW TO TAKE YOUR PULSE

Immediately upon stopping your workout, take your pulse for 10 seconds in order to calculate the training effect. Then multiply by six and you'll have calculated your actual heart rate.

HOW TO EXERCISE YOUR HEART

The first thing to do is decide which kind of aerobic activity you want to do. Good examples are walking, bicycling, swimming, jogging, cross-country skiing, rowing and rope jumping.

How *hard* should you do it? Most experts feel that to achieve a training effect you must exercise at an intensity which will allow your heart to beat between 60 and 80 percent of your maximum capacity.

To compute your maximum capacity or heart rate, use this formula:

Use the number 220, and subtract your age.

$$220 - (\text{your age}) = \text{maximum}$$

A mid-range training rate zone for your heart could be figured out by calculating 70% of your maximum.

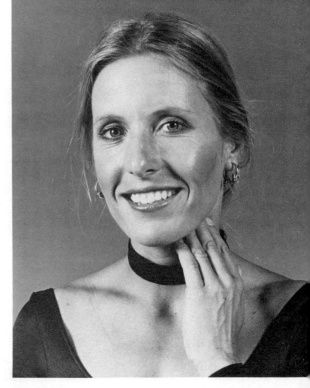

For example:
If you are 40 years old,

$$220 - 40 = 180$$

$$70\% \text{ of } 180 = 126 \text{ beats per minute}$$

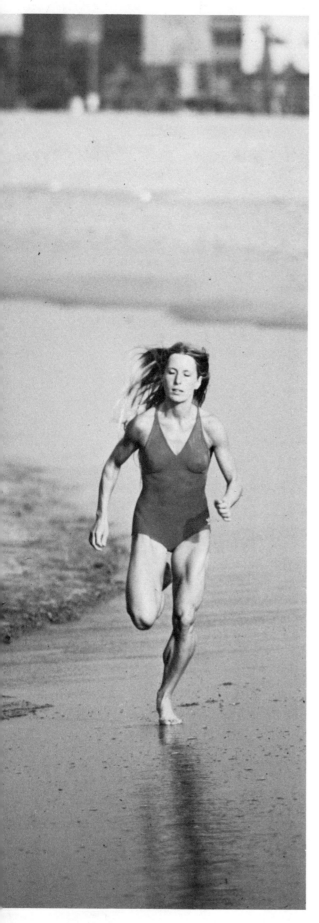

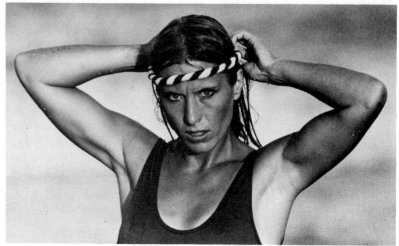

For convenience, compute how many beats that would mean for 10 seconds—the number is 21.

Now you can take your heart rate for 10 seconds during your workout and know if you're working hard enough.

As your cardiovascular system becomes stronger, your work will become easier and you will be forced to increase the tempo or intensity of your activities to maintain a training effect on your heart. This is similar to the way a 10-pound dumbbell can become too light for your biceps once you become stronger.

How Long?

The absolute minimum duration is 10 minutes. Fifteen to 20 minutes of honest aerobic activity per day is considered to be very good. Of course, this will not get you into the Olympics, but it will certainly keep you in good shape. Spend a few minutes before your workout by doing some easy activity as a warm-up, and a few minutes at the conclusion of the workout as a cool-down.

How Often?

Naturally, how often depends upon how intensely and how long you exercise. The general rule is that 4 workouts per week are better than 3, and that 5 are better than 4. If you can only exercise 3 times a week, then increase the length of each session by 5 to 10 minutes and do the workouts on alternate days. Two workouts a week are better than 1, but not effective enough for training your heart, although you can maintain a minimum standard of fitness this way.

Making Time

1. Set a regular time for your exercise and let nothing else keep you from this appointment.

2. Find a workout partner if possible. It's more fun, and it's more difficult to miss when someone else is depending on you.

3. Use good equipment. A beautiful leotard or super-comfortable shoes also make you feel good.

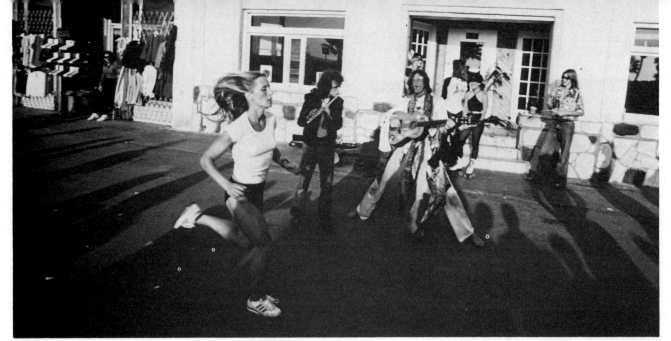

Venice Beach, California

WHAT YOU CAN EXPECT FROM GETTING INTO SHAPE

1. A better shape—a firmer body.
2. A release from stress and negative energy.
3. Better posture.
4. More energy, vitality.
5. Self-respect.
6. Improved circulation.
7. Better sleep.
8. Better resistance to disease.
9. Good eating habits.
10. A calmer, more positive outlook.
11. Weight loss if overweight.
12. Compliments from your friends and neighbors.

WALKING

There are no special rules for walking. Just put on a pair of comfortable shoes and go to it. Strive for good posture and allow your arms to swing freely. Walkers experience fewer foot and leg problems than runners or joggers, and there is always the added advantage of being able to see more scenery because of the slower speed.

Taking Fido with you is a good idea, but *only* if he's trained to stay with you. Kids can be pushed in a stroller, and very young babies can be taken along papoose style in a baby backpack.

Program

- Start with 20 minutes a day (about 1¼ miles).
- Do this for one week.
- Increase by 5 minutes per week until you reach 45–60 minutes a day.
- Maintain this until you can do this easily, then try "resistance walking"—uphill, or in soft sand or deep snow.

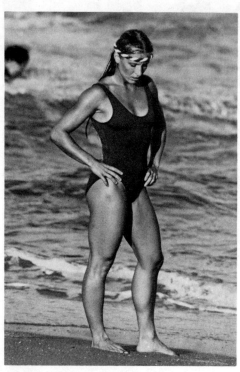

After a swim in the Atlantic

Tips

- Don't worry about distance, just be sure to walk briskly for the time allowed.
- Try to walk to and from work.
- If you live too far, park or get off the bus 40 minutes of walking time away from the office or factory. Then walk in.
- If you live close to work, take a roundabout route.
- You can use the same principle for grocery shopping—wheel a collapsible shopping cart with you.

SWIMMING

Advantages
- Uses all the major muscles.
- The water's buoyancy factor takes pressure off joints.

Disadvantages
- Requires a pool, ocean, or lake, and the ability to swim.

Workout # 1

A. Swim slowly one pool length with breast stroke or sidestroke.
B. Using a kickboard, flutter kick for 5 minutes.
C. Swim 1 length with front stroke. Return with breast stroke. Repeat for 8 minutes.
D. Kick for 2 minutes as a warm-down.

Workout #2

A. Flutter kick for 5 minutes.
B. Swim 2 lengths (out and back) with front stroke. Swim 1 length with breast stroke. Repeat for 15 minutes.
C. Float on your back, kicking only for 5 minutes.

Workout #3

A. "Dolphin" kick with kickboard for 5 minutes. This is a type of kick where you pretend your feet are tied together at the ankles, and you kick both legs at the same time.
B. Swim with front stroke for 15 minutes.
C. Flutter kick with kickboard for 5 minutes.

Workout #4

A. Swim with backstroke for 5 minutes.
B. Swim with frontstroke for 15 minutes, pushing your pace, or "surging," every third length.
C. Dolphin kick for ten minutes.

Occasionally try climbing out of the pool after the workout and then doing a racing dive or two, continuing for a whole lap—really go for it! Have someone time you.

EXERCISE BICYCLE

Advantages
- Can be used indoors in all weather.
- You can listen to your favorite music.

Disadvantages
- You must be creative in your workouts to keep them from becoming stale.

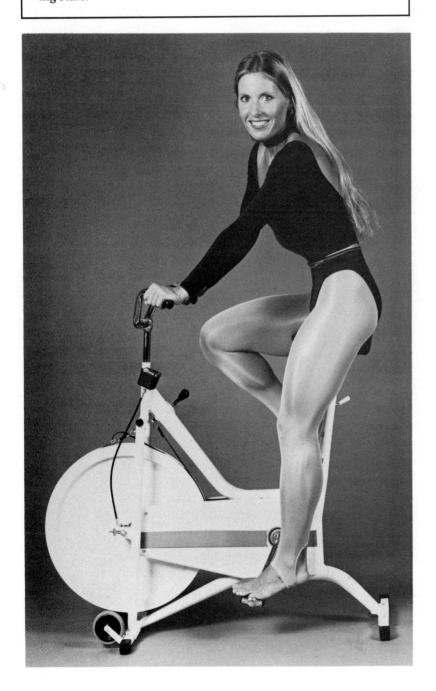

Tips

Be sure to adjust seat correctly.
Keep a chart handy next to the bike listing your "world records."

•

Workout #1

A. Two minutes easy pedaling with no resistance.
B. Eight minutes pedaling with resistance. Check heart rate several times to ensure it is beating within your training zone.
C. Three minutes backward pedaling.
D. Continue for 1 week, and then increase Part B 30 seconds a day to a total of 12 minutes. Now you are ready for Workout #2.

Workout #2

A. Two minutes easy pedaling warm-up.
B. Steady resistance pedaling for 5 minutes.
C. Then, once every minute for 10 minutes, pedal faster for 20 strokes (a stroke is counted every time the left foot goes down).
D. Backward pedaling for 5 minutes.

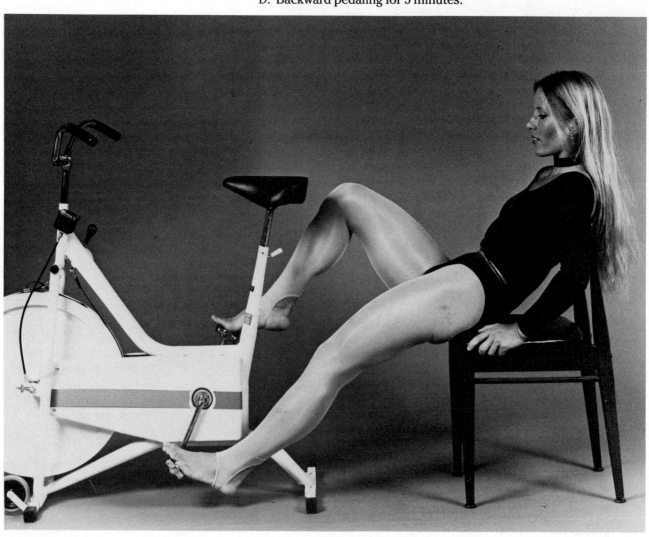

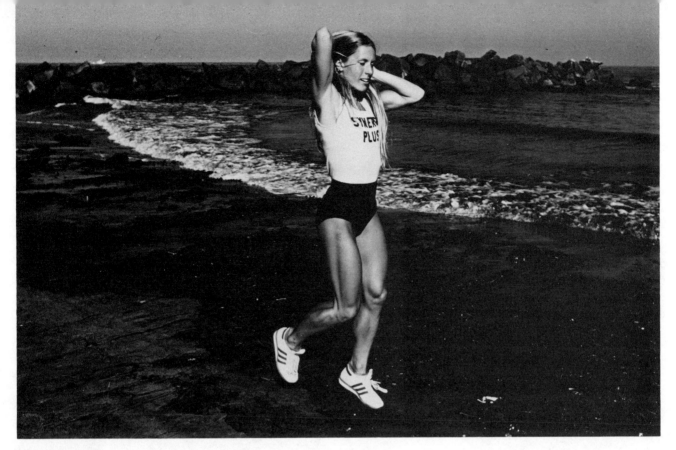

Workout #3

A. Two minutes easy pedaling warm-up.
B. Workout #2, Part C.
C. Ten minutes of steady-pace pedaling while sitting in a chair *(figure I)*.
D. Three minutes backward pedaling. *Note:* If your stationary bicycle does not offer resistance while you are pedaling backward, then substitute chair cycling. Backward pedaling and chair cycling benefit the upper portion of the backs of your thighs.

Workout #4

A. Two minutes easy pedaling warm-up.
B. Ten minutes steady pace with resistance, keeping your heart rate in the training zone.
C. Try for a one-minute "world record," seeing how far on the odometer you can go for this time.
D. Increase your world record timed distances by 30 seconds each week until you reach 20 minutes.
E. *Variation:* Try standing up on the pedals—pedaling without sitting on the bicycle seat.

Tips

You must check your heat rate and adjust the tension so that you can keep your heart beating within your training zone.

Put on some great music and go crazy!

Change the location of the bicycle—on a balcony if your apartment has one. Or, put it in your bathroom, wear your bikini and turn all the hot water faucets on and pretend you are in the Tropics.

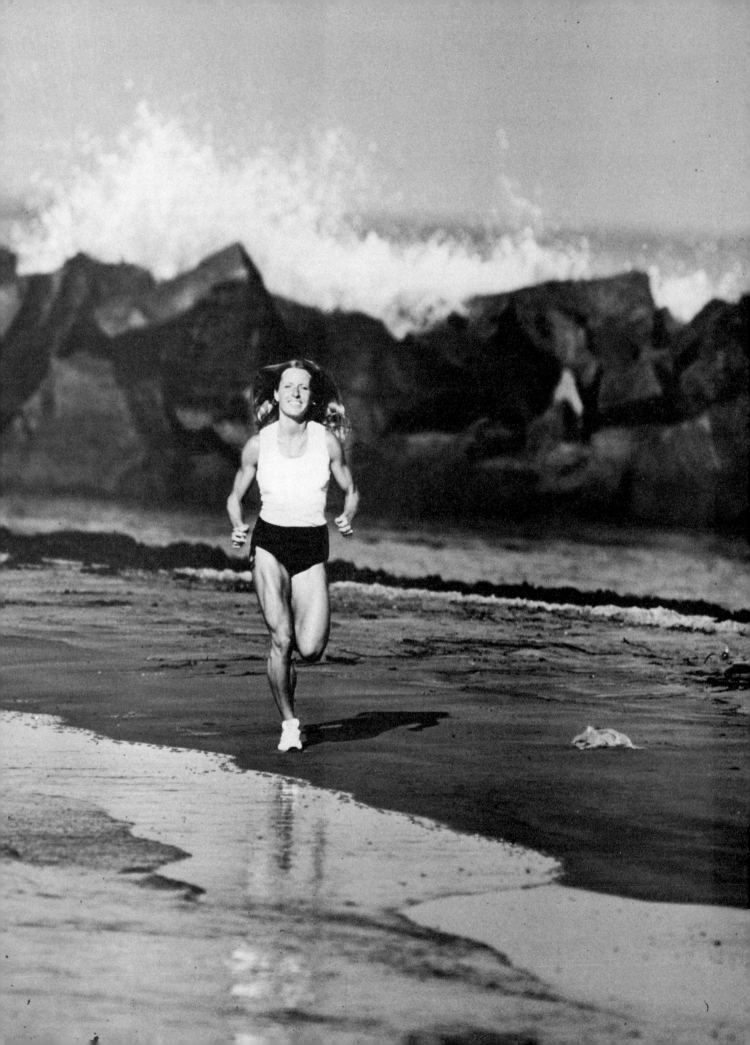

RUNNING

10-K FEVER

On any given weekend in North America, chances are that there is a 10-K (6.2 mile) race taking place somewhere near you. And with it, an infectiously festive atmosphere that's impossible to resist.

Marching bands, balloons and crazy costumes are often part of the parade, except that the crowds you see standing around all *become* the parade once the gun goes off. Then you'll see grandparents, kids, parents and what seems like all their friends and neighbors all running like crazy down the street. Some races have 30,000 or more participants.

Of course, there are the "stallions" at the front of the horde, whose ranks eventually dwindle down to the first female and first male winner. But there are usually prizes as well for the top finishers in age categories that can start from ten years and under and proceed in five-year increments all the way up to eighty years and older. These age categories have caused an interesting phenomenon among the more than forty million runners on the continent: they can't wait to get older and into the next age category so that their chances of winning will be increased. I've known more than a few thirty-nine-year-olds who have gone into "secret training" for one year. Then, with the birthday cake barely digested, they make a big comeback race to cap honors in the 40 or over division.

10-K is a good challenge which requires a fair amount of preparation if you are to enjoy the race. Yet it's not as depleting or arduous as a marathon (26.2 miles), which, incidentally, I don't recommend for anybody's health. Before starting the following plan, you will need from four to eight weeks of time (depending on your level of fitness) to get to the point where you can jog nonstop for twenty minutes, four times a week.

HOW TO RUN YOUR FIRST 10-K

The chart is designed for every runner or aspiring runner. The race is six weeks away, and the program is suitable for anyone of good health. (Be sure to get a medical check-up.) For those who are already runners, skip the first weeks, as you see fit. Remember that you should never run in pain, and the best way to ensure that is to stretch before and after every workout.

On race day, be sure to jog five minutes before the start and keep moving. Take advantage of water stations; get used to drinking during your training runs.

Regardless of your training, you will find the race momentum can pull you along faster than you anticipated. Don't get carried away. You don't want to go too fast at the beginning and deplete your energy before the last leg of the race.

The first fact to remember about any race is that it should be fun —the same thing goes for training. Enjoy yourself, and keep in mind that running is a test of athletics, not heroics.

	SUN	MON	TUES	WED	THURS	FRI	SAT
WEEK ONE	Jog 1 mi, easy pace	Brisk 30-min walk*	Jog 15 min	Run 1 mi, steady pace	Run 20 min, steady pace	Brisk 45-min walk	Jog 20 min
WEEK TWO	2–3 mi run, steady pace	20-min jog, easy pace	20-min run, stretch, speed work**	30-min jog	3-mile run, steady pace; try harder last 10 min	Brisk 45-min walk	Jog 20 min
WEEK THREE	3–4 mi run, steady pace	20-min jog, easy pace	20-min run, stretch, speed work	30-min jog	35-min run, steady pace; try harder last 10 min	Brisk 45-min walk	Jog 30 min
WEEK FOUR	4–5 mi run; get used to drinking water	20-min jog, easy pace	20-min run, stretch, speed work	30-min jog	40-min run, steady pace; try harder last 10 min	Brisk 60-min walk	Jog 30 min
WEEK FIVE	5-mi run	20-min jog, easy pace	20-min run, stretch, speed work	30-min jog	40-min run, steady pace; try harder last 10 min	Brisk 60-min walk	Jog 30 min
WEEK SIX	5-mi run	20-min jog, easy pace	20-min run, stretch, speed work	20-min jog	30-min walk	Rest	Jog 10 min

* Don't laugh at my advice to walk. Walking strengthens the feet (especially if you walk on the sand), and it gets you used to spending time on them.

** Speed work consists of 10-minute segments of jogging, running and walking after you run. Use the distance between telephone poles as your guide. The first week of speed work consists of jogging the distance (between 3 telephone poles, say), then running the distance hard, then walking it; repeat the sequence. For the second week, double the distance for the jog/run portion; the third week, triple it; the fourth and fifth weeks, quadruple it. The walk portion always stays the same.

MARATHON MANIA

In 490 B.C. a lone Greek named Pheidippides ran from Marathon to Athens to announce the news of the Athenian victory over the invading Persians. He ran the twenty-five miles, gasped "Rejoice, we have conquered" and then dropped dead on the spot.

Three thousand, three hundred and eighty-six years later, more than 60,000 people lined the streets of Athens to cheer for Spiridon Loues, the winner of the world's first staged marathon. He ran a tough twenty-five mile race in 2:58:50 to become the first modern day Olympic champion.

Spiridon was a humble water carrier from Marousi, Greece, but today millions of people have run the updated 26.2-mile event—male and female—from every walk of life.

Completing the marathon is seen as "graduate school" for the millions of runners and joggers in North America. While finishing the event can be an incredibly exhilarating experience if you are prepared for it, too often the novice runner enters a marathon with a lot of heart, and not enough training.

Even in the Boston Marathon where participants must run a strict qualifying time to enter, almost one of every five starters never makes it to the finish.

The marathon is a challenge—a tough one to resist—but one that must be faced with equal amounts of courage and preparation. To ignore this is to invite injury.

My advice to future marathoners is to run in 10-K races for a year, entering one every two to three weeks, then going for some over-distance twenty-mile runs on the off weeks. Think of increasing your weekly mileage over the years rather than over the months.

For instance, if you're doing forty miles a week now, think of upping that to fifty next year, sixty the year after, seventy the year after that. Wait until you are doing sixty or seventy quality miles a week with speed training as well before doing your first marathon.

Then the marathon itself will be a good experience for you—unlike the rather final event it was for Pheidippides in 490 B.C.

PUMPING AIR AND PUMPING IRON

- Keep track of your workouts in a little notebook.
- Warm-up before each workout by brisk walking, running on the spot, skipping rope or something of this nature for five minutes. Then do the stretches listed at the end of each body-part section.
- Feel free to change around the workouts to different days, but try to allow a hard day–easy day combination.
- Do some stomach exercises every day.

THE CHART						
Sunday	Monday	Tuesday	Wednesday	Thursday	Friday	Saturday
Longest workout: Do 2 x your usual average, run, walk, swim or bike ride	Easy aerobic workout (1/3 of Sunday's) Weights: Stomach, arms and shoulders, derrière	Speed day intervals— Time yourself over short distances Runners—see 10K chart Swimmers, bikers, walkers— see your section for examples	A steady paced medium effort Aerobic workout (½ of Sunday's)	Easy aerobic workout Weights: Stomach Back Chest Legs	R E S T	Speed day (See Tuesday)

EXERCISE AND CALORIES

Activity	Approximate Calories Used			
	1 hr	½ hr	¼ hr	5 mins
Walking (slow, 2 mph)	150	75	38	13
Walking (medium, 3 mph)	300	150	75	25
Walking (fast, 5 mph)	480	240	120	40
Golf (with power cart)	200	100	50	17
Golf (carrying bag)	360	180	90	30
Typical housework	300	150	75	25
Scrubbing floors	360	180	90	30
Bowling	300	150	75	25
Bicycling (slow, 6 mph)	300	150	75	25
Bicycling (medium, 8 mph)	400	200	100	33
Bicycling (fast)	600	300	150	50
Tennis (doubles)	360	180	90	30
Tennis (singles)	480	240	120	40
Ice/Roller skating	420	210	105	35
Jogging (slow, 5 mph)	600	300	150	50
Running (medium, 6 mph)	700	350	175	58
Skiing (downhill)	600	300	150	50
Lawn mowing (power mower)	250	125	63	21
Lawn mowing (hand mower)	300	150	75	25
Swimming (medium)	400	200	100	33

These figures are approximate and calculated for a 150-lb. person

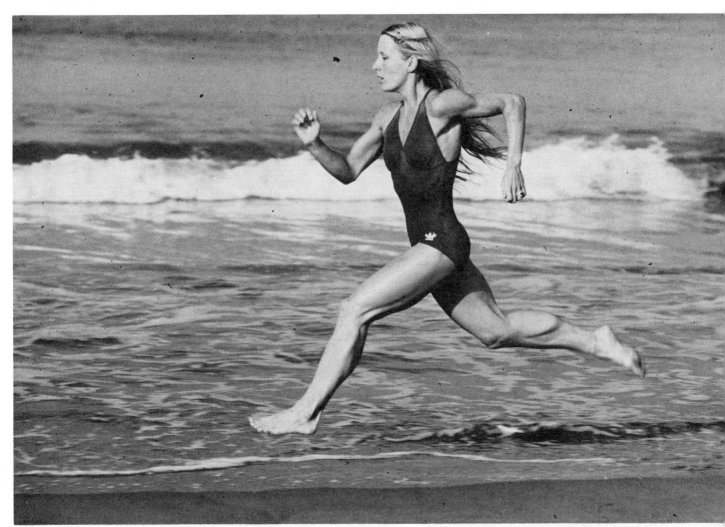

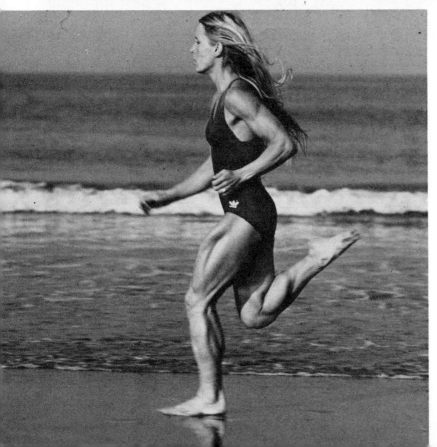

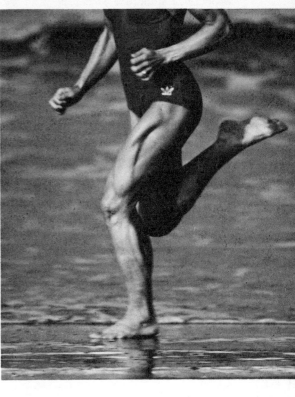

EXERCISE CHART FOR CHEATERS

Figures are based on data for a 150-lb. person, so lighter or heavier people will use fewer or more calories accordingly. An athlete in excellent condition will also use fewer calories due to oxygen efficiency. Figures are approximate and are based on information from USDA food charts.

Food	Weight 1 oz = 28,349 grams	Calories	Walking	Bicycling	Swimming	Jogging
	gm	kcal	min	min	min	min
Asparagus, cooked, 4 spears	60	10	2	2	1	1
Angel food cake, 1 pc (¹⁄₁₂ of 10″ cake)	53	135	26	20	16	14
Apple, raw, 1 med (2½″ diam)	150	87	17	13	10	9
Almonds, dried, salted, 12–15 nuts	15	93	18	14	11	9
Almond bar, chocolate, 1 bar (1¼ oz)	38	310	60	46	36	31
Blue Cheese (Roquefort) dressing	14	70	14	10	8	7
Bacon, lettuce, tomato sandwich—1 white toasted	148	282	54	42	34	28
Bologna with mayonnaise, sandwich 1 slice; tsp	68	220	42	33	26	22
Beer, 8 oz glass	240	115	22	18	14	12
Bread (fresh & toasted) (white, rye, whole wheat, Italian, French), 1 slice	23	60	12	9	7	6
Bread, buttered, 1 slice, 1 pat	28	96	18	15	11	10
Biscuit, honey, 2″ diam; 1 pat; 1 tsp	40	164	32	25	19	16
Bacon, crisp fried, 2 strips (20 strips/lb)	15	90	17	14	11	9
Banana split	300	594	114	89	71	59
Banana, 1 med	150	127	24	19	15	13
Beef TV dinner	310	350	67	52	42	35
Broccoli, 1 stalk (5½″)	100	32	6	5	4	3
Cauliflower, cooked, drained, ⅛ cup	105	31	6	5	4	3
Corn, sweet, canned, ½ cup	128	85	16	13	10	9
Chicken TV dinner, fried	310	542	104	81	65	54
Chicken noodle soup	240	62	12	10	7	6
Caramel, 1 oz	30	118	23	18	14	12
Chocolate milk, teacup (6½ oz)	200	210	40	32	25	21
Coca-Cola, 8 oz glass	240	105	20	16	12	11
Coffee & sugar, 1 cup; 1 tsp	200	30	6	5	4	3
Chili con carne, no beans, 1 cup	250	334	64	50	40	33
Chicken breast, broiled, ½ breast (no bone)	72	105	20	16	13	11
Chicken breast, fried, ½ breast (no bone)	76	155	29	23	19	16
Cupcake with icing, 1 (2½″ diam)	36	130	25	20	16	13
Cottage cheese, 1 round tbs	30	30	6	4	4	3
Cheese, American, 1 slice (1 oz)	30	112	22	17	13	11
Cheese, toasted sandwich	85	286	55	43	34	29
Cheeseburger	180	462	89	69	55	46
Doughnut, 1 average	32	125	24	19	15	13
Egg, fried or scrambled, 1 med: 1 tsp oil	53	108	21	16	13	11
Fruit cocktail, ½ cup, water pack	100	37	7	6	4	4
French dressing	14	57	11	9	7	6
Frankfurter (1 frank 8/lb pkg)	56	170	32	26	20	17
Grapefruit juice, ½ glass (4 oz)	120	47	9	7	6	5
Hamburger, cooked, 1 patty (3″ diam x 1″)	85	224	43	34	27	22

Food	Weight 1 oz = 28,349 grams	Calories	Walking	Bicycling	Swimming	Jogging
	gm	kcal	min	min	min	min
Hamburger	150	350	57	52	42	35
Hot dog with ketchup	110	258	50	39	31	26
Italian dressing	14	100	19	15	12	10
Ice cream—1 scoop	60	115	22	17	14	12
Ice cream bar, choc. coated, 1 bar	60	195	37	30	23	20
Lettuce, iceberg, ⅛ head (4¾″ diam)	55	10	2	2	1	1
Low calorie dressing	14	15	3	2	2	1
Lobster, boiled with butter; 2 tbs butter	334	308	59	46	37	31
Mayonnaise	14	100	19	15	12	10
Milk, whole, 8 oz glass	240	160	31	25	19	16
Martini, cocktail, 3½ oz	100	140	27	22	16	14
Meatloaf TV dinner	310	370	71	56	44	37
Mushrooms, fried, 4 med	70	78	15	12	9	8
Melba toast, unsalted, 1 thin slice	4	15	3	2	2	2
Milk, buttermilk, 8 oz glass	240	88	17	13	10	9
Orange, raw, 1 med (3″ diam)	150	73	14	11	9	7
Orange juice, ½ glass (4 oz)	120	54	10	8	6	5
Pork chops, lean, 2 chops (3 oz cooked)	90	260	49	39	31	26
Peanuts, roasted, 6–8 nuts	15	86	17	13	10	9
Peanuts, dry roasted, 8–10 nuts	16	80	15	12	10	8
Pretzels, 3 ring, 4 (148/lb)	12	48	9	7	6	5
Popsicle	95	70	4	10	8	7
Pancake, 4″ diam	45	105	20	16	12	11
Pancake & syrup, 4″ diam; 2 tbs	85	204	39	31	24	20
Peach with cottage cheese; 2 med halves; 2 tbs cheese	156	105	20	16	13	10
Potato salad, ½ cup	100	99	19	15	12	10
Peanut butter and jelly; 1 rounded tbs; 1 level tbs	86	290	55	45	35	29
Pizza, sausage, ⅛ of 14″ dia pie	75	195	38	29	23	20
Peas, green, cooked, ½ cup	80	58	11	9	7	6
Potato, baked with butter, 1 med; 2 pats	110	160	31	24	19	16
Raisin, dried; 1 tbs	10	30	6	4	4	3
Sunflower seeds, 30–40 nuts	15	84	16	13	10	8
Shrimp, French fried, 3½ oz	100	225	43	34	27	23
Tomato soup	245	90	17	14	11	9
Turkey, roasted, 2 slices; (3″ x 3½″)	80	160	31	24	19	16
Turkey, roasted with gravy, 2 slices; 2 tbs	115	240	46	36	29	24
Tomato, tuna salad, 1 med; 2 tbs	180	100	19	15	12	10
T-bone steak, broiled, 3 oz cooked	90	175	33	26	21	18
Waffle, plain, 5½″ diam	120	345	66	52	41	35
Watermelon, 1 wedge (4″ x 8″)	10	30	6	4	4	3

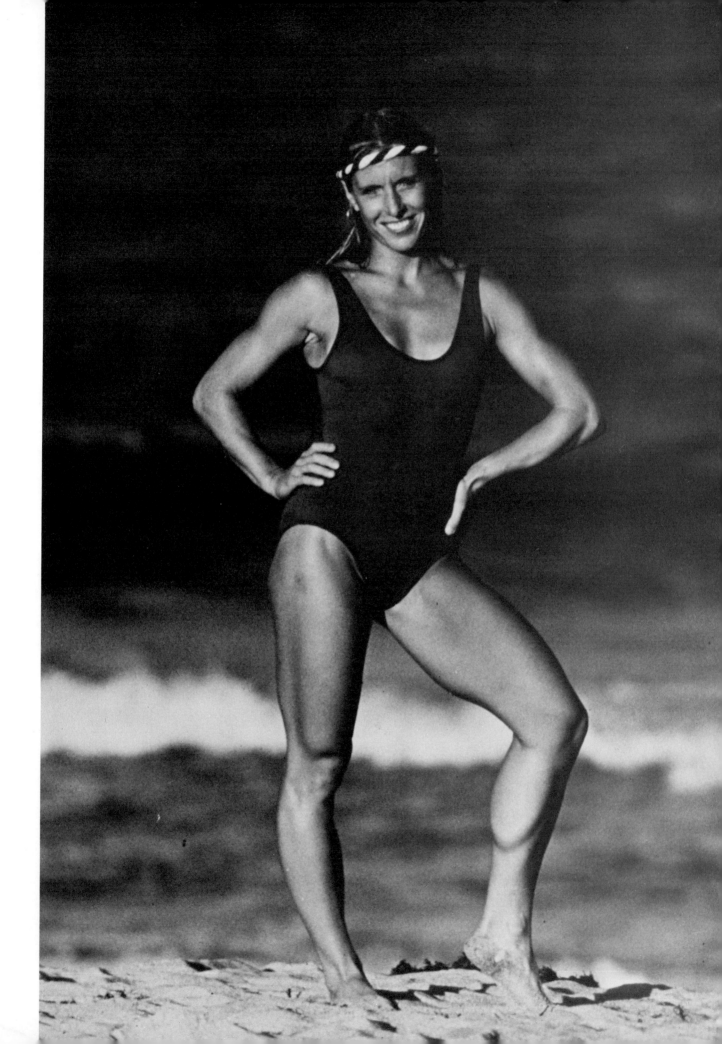

4
STAYING WITH IT

HERBAL REMEDIES

Getting stronger requires a certain flexing of mental muscles as well as those you may have forgotten about on other parts of your body.

But in order to *stay with it,* sometimes you need a little help from outside sources. The stresses of everyday life, the draining effect of a long winter, even the good honest ache of worked muscles can sabotage the best of intentions when you're trying to continue getting stronger day after day.

This is where sweet relief may be provided by rediscovery of the herbal remedies handed down through the ages.

In 570 B.C. Nebuchadnezzar had flower beds of fragrant herbs planted in the famous Hanging Gardens of Babylon so that breezes could spread the perfume far and wide.

Roman soldiers added mugwort to their baths to relieve sore and aching muscles caused by their long marches, and Cleopatra was said to preserve her beauty with honey facials.

History and legend shows that we have always derived great pleasure and relief from the delicate scents of aromatic herbs and flowers.

There *are* alternatives to the drugs which are so pushed on athletes today. There *are* other pick-me-ups than coffee, doughnuts and cigarettes. There is no rule that states the evening must begin with a martini, or that you have to pay someone a lot of money for fancy skin creams and cosmetics full of chemicals.

I don't believe in aspirin, coffee or mood-altering drugs. I believe that nature has a remedy for all of our self-induced maladies, and that we must be patient in our quest to become stronger—allowing our body to choose the rate it needs to heal. Why must we egotistically contrive a cause and effect with drugs that could be short-lived and have possible harmful side effects for the future?

This is why I have studied herbs. I have become wary of publicity-conscious "healers" waving hypodermic needles, claiming they can heal the body. The body heals itself—often in spite of our interference.

Don't expect overnight miracle cures from using herbs, or you'll be disappointed. And avoid the "If *this* much is good for me, then *twice* that must *really* be good for me" type of mentality.

However, when you need a little help from a friend to get you by, or when your commitment to getting stronger needs bolstering, then a garden of earthly delights is waiting for you. Herbs are nature's gifts to us, to be used with prudence and understanding.

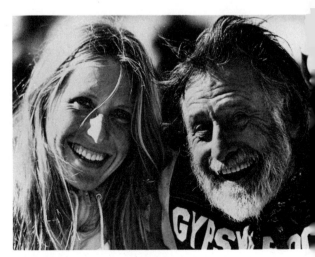

With world-famous naturalist Gypsy Boots

95

HEADACHE

Nutmeg often shows up in hangover recipes, yet the aroma itself soothes a headache. Grate nutmeg into a flame or on the stove burner, but be sure to use small doses. This herb can have narcotic effects if used in excess.

SUPERSTAR PAIN RELIEVER

Of course, extreme or persistent pain of any kind requires immediate attention by your physician. But for everyday headaches, menstrual cramps, and the like, the following method can offer enormous relief of pain in five to seven minutes.

Rub an ice cube on the hand, about one inch in from the webbing between the thumb and index finger as shown on page 152. Apply for ten minutes, or until the ice cube melts.

FOLKLORE'S FAMOUS HERBAL TEAS FOR WHAT AILS YOU

Folklore medicine has raised the use of herbal teas to an art form. Historical references to herbal teas have survived in ancient documents, and more recently it seems everyone has or knows someone who has a grandmother who made teas from flowers or leaves.

Today, herbal teas are no longer the domain of little old ladies who crochet in front of a wood stove. Specialty teas are coming back into style, complete with "flow thru" tea bags, fancy boxes and advertising campaigns to match.

These commercial brews are really more for pleasurable sipping, however, and are not meant for relief from "what ails you" in the traditional sense. They are a marvelous alternative to the caffeine and chemicals of coffee, black tea and soft drinks, so be sure to sample a few brews before trying to pick a favorite. A real tip-off to the taste of the tea is the scent—that is, if you like the smell, chances are you'll like the taste.

The teas listed here are home brews that different cultures have used throughout history for the various non-crisis aches and pains. Drugs and doctors were for life-threatening situations only.

Before aspirin tablets, for instance, white willow bark was steeped in boiling water—a process which chemists now realize as one that extracts salicin from the bark, the basis for aspirin.

Those faint of heart were given decoction of foxglove, a small plant with purple flowers that grows by roadsides. In present times, foxglove is known by part of its botanical name, digitalis, the famous heart medicine.

Botanists now propagate pink periwinkle blossoms for the two superstar anticancer drugs, vincristine and vinblastine. Mayapple blossoms yield drugs for brain tumors and Hodgkin's disease. The Incas of Mexico gathered dioscorea, a wild yam which supplies substances for birth control pills.

How many more of these undiscovered or forgotten superstar plants are crushed by bulldozers as forests are cleared, or suffocated by herbicides that we relentlessly spray on our lands? Perhaps teaching our children the value of the plants beneath our feet will not only ease their immediate aches and pains, but provide for the health of generations of our children's children to come.

How to Make a Fine Cup of Herbal Tea

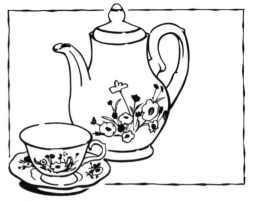

Use one generous teaspoon of your favorite tea to two cups of water. Bring the water to a rapid boil in a glass or enamel pot, remove from heat and add the herbs. Let stand for five minutes. Strain it and serve either hot or cold. Honey may be used to flavor and the tea may be refrigerated for use throughout the day.

Folklore's Top Twenty Herbal Teas

1. *Anemia*	—Cayenne, comfrey, dandelion
2. *Arthritic pains*	—Chaparral, alfalfa, valerian root
3. *Constipation*	—Senna, flaxseed
4. *Diarrhea*	—Barberry bark, slippery elm
5. *Digestion*	—Ginger, peppermint, fenugreek
6. *Endurance*	—Capsicum, ginseng, bee pollen
7. *Flatulence*	—Peppermint
8. *Headache*	—Ginger, catnip, chamomile
(Nervous headache)	—Lavender blossoms
9. *Indigestion*	—Ginger, papaya seeds, catnip
10. *Impotence*	—Damiana
11. *Insomnia*	—Hops, chamomile, passion flower
12. *Mental Fatigue*	—Ginseng, gotu kola, fo-ti tieng, comfrey
13. *Menstrual cramps*	—Valerian root, ginger
14. *Muscle cramps*	—Chaparral, comfrey, dandelion, alfalfa
15. *Pain*	—Scullcap, hops, valerian root, catnip
16. *Scar Tissue on Skin*	—Marigold, marshmallow root, slippery elm, lemon and honey
17. *Skin (Acne)*	—Oat straw, chaparral, dandelion, sassafras
18. *Throat (sore)*	—Ginger, slippery elm, lemon and honey
19. *Tonic*	—Licorice root, dandelion, laurel
20. *Vitality*	—Ginseng, gotu kola, licorice root

SKIN

The following recipes are for active people—who need skin care more than anyone. Life in the sunlight can just dry it out.

Some athletes have slender, sinewy bodies, but wrinkled, weather-beaten hands and faces. You don't *have* to look like this. The increased oxygen uptake because of aerobic exercise increases the body's demand for antioxidants, the same elements that prevent rust on a piece of metal.

Vitamin C is important in this regard, too. It is involved in the manufacture of collagen protein in the body—the tissue cement of cells. It prevents bruises and excess scarring and is essential for our skin membranes inside and out.

Minerals, of course, especially silicon, calcium and sulphur, are important for healthy skin and hair, and who could forget the adage "Take zinc. Don't stink"? Zinc is invaluable for skin, hair and nails, is an antioxidant, and seems to prevent body odor.

Of concern to athletes is the fact that Vitamin E has also been linked in studies by Dr. Evan Shute with oxygen uptake. So being sure of an adequate supply could mean better performances and fewer wrinkles!

BRUISES

Vitamin C should be increased if you seem to bruise easily. This formula is to help remove discoloration.

1 part cayenne pepper
1 part glycerine

"Rescue" by the Fort Lauderdale Beach Patrol: Erik Jersted (far left) and Chuck Niessen (far right), world record holders in ocean rowing

Mix. Apply with cotton balls.
    Caution: Avoid eyes and mucous membranes!

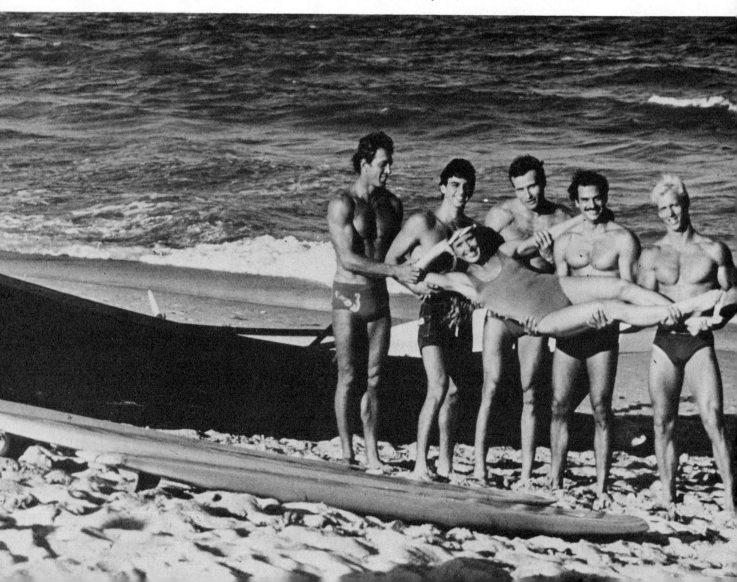

OATMEAL FACIAL

This is good for blemishes, and combination oily/dry skin.

¼ cup ground oatmeal
(you can use quick 1 minute
type of oats)

2 tsp honey
1 tsp milk

Blend the honey and oatmeal well. If it seems too thick and un-wieldy, add the milk. Apply to clean face and neck, avoiding the eye area. Leave it on 30 to 40 minutes, and lay down with your feet up if you can. I've made this facial with just milk and oatmeal, heating the whole thing in a small enamel pot or double boiler first.

Caution: If you do the milk and oatmeal recipe, do *not* laugh while it's drying. It will feel like your face will crack!

After half an hour, use a washcloth with warm water to help you remove the facial. Finish with an astringent or witch hazel.

ATHLETE'S FOOT

Sprinkle garlic powder on affected areas. Your feet will smell like a pizza, but garlic banished a pesky bout of athlete's foot for me once —never to return. You can sprinkle a little in your socks, too.

Apple cider vinegar is another home remedy for athlete's foot. Apply generously to affected areas several times a day, using cotton balls. Allow to dry before wearing clean socks.

SUNBURN AND OTHER BURNS
(including JELLYFISH STINGS)

Aloe Vera

Aloe Vera has been used by different cultures for thousands of years, and it is known all over the world by its scientific name. It can survive long periods of drought, and when one leaf is cut off, the plant heals quickly, growing in another direction. Aloe Vera is used externally for burns, rashes and cuts, and internally for ulcers, colitis and a host of other maladies including flatulence and indigestion. It is also valuable as a skin moisturizer when applied with cotton balls.

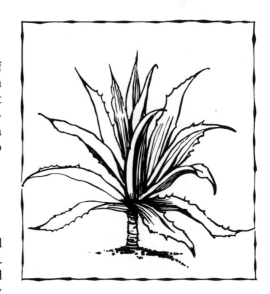

Aloe Vera Juice

Squeeze directly from the leaves onto the skin. If using bottled pure aloe vera gel, apply with cotton balls. Reapply every half hour. You will see how the skin seems to just "drink it in." For jellyfish and man-of-war stings, I use alcohol first, then apply the aloe vera gel by splitting the leaf in long sections and gently wrapping pieces right onto the skin with gauze or an Ace bandage. Change frequently.

BURNING FEET

Basketball and tennis players often get "hot spots" on their feet, which are red, burning areas, usually under a callous, that come from the constant friction of lateral movement.

4–8 large very ripe tomatoes (if your feet are over size 10, you'll need more)
⅓ cup water

Throw it all in a blender and blend until liquefied. If you prefer a cold foot soak, add crushed ice and use as is. (The "snow" on your refrigerator freezer does nicely instead of crushed ice.) Otherwise, heat mixture until it is slightly hotter than bath water temperature. Pour in a basin and stick your feet in for 10 to 15 minutes. One of the basketball players I coached said he puts the tomatoes back on the stove after that and makes spaghetti sauce out of it, but that is certainly up to you. If you decide to go this route, however, I do suggest you refrain from telling your guests.

ANOINT YOUR CROWNING GLORY

A beautiful head of hair is an asset to anyone, male or female. Yet hot showers, saunas, constant sunshine, the hot studio lights, ocean spray and even jet travel really give my hair a beating. And with hair down to my waist, there's a lot of it to look after.

A very kind elderly woman from Paris first mixed up this hair ointment for me. She recalled a time more than half a century ago when as a young girl she had worn her hair down to her waist. Her mother had shown her how to care for her hair this way—after applying the mixture, shampooing with castile soap, and then finishing with a rinse of chamomile tea to assure the blond highlights.

My hair seems to absolutely thrive on this formula, and I hope yours does, too. I use it at least once a month.

1 cup honey
¼ cup olive oil
¼ cup almond oil

Mix ingredients a few days before you intend to use it, and store at room temperature. No need to refrigerate. Shake well before using.

Really massage this thoroughly into your hair and scalp. Leave it on at least thirty minutes. I often leave it on for an hour or longer. Be careful about going outside with this on your hair—bees, wasps and all kinds of insect creatures will go wild over you. (You catch more flies with honey, as they say.) Wash with your favorite shampoo.

SOAP

Of course, use some in the obvious places daily. However, there is no need to lather yourself up all over as they do in the commercials. Soap dries your skin if overused. Pick one that is not full of chemicals and preservatives. As in food shopping, read labels. Chances are that if you can't pronounce it, you don't need it. Some deodorant soaps contain ingredients which can cause reactions to the sun like blistering or blotchiness in sensitive people. Old-fashioned castile soap used sparingly will work fine for most people. Natural food stores also sell gentle, fragrance-free alternatives to chemical suds.

HERBAL BATHS

Luxuriating in a bathtub and inhaling the steamy fragrance of sweet herbs is surely one of life's pleasures that is deserved after a hard day of exercise. You need a muslin bag or a large square of soft mesh material for the herbs. Mix all the herbs together loosely in the bag, tie the top securely and then place in the tub. Pour on the hottest water that comes out of the tap—enough to cover the bag—and let soak for 10 minutes. Then fill the tub the usual way and climb in. You deserve it! Think virtuous thoughts.

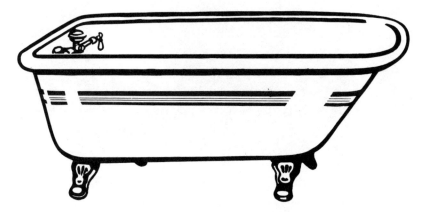

For Relaxing Nerves and Sore Muscles:

1 handful dried lavender flowers
1 handful rosemary leaves
1 handful dried chamomile flowers
1 handful mint leaves

Any single one of the above or any combination of the above could be tried. Use triple amounts for single herb baths.

MASSAGE OIL

Caution: Keep oils away from eyes and mucous membranes!

1 cup sweet almond oil
4–5 drops of an aromatic oil of your choice (even vanilla extract is very nice)
(Baby oil is often used by some for massage but it is usually 100% mineral oil, which is toxic to the body.)

The only direction for this formula is: apply with caring hands to the tired body of a deserving athlete. Other oils with a deep penetrating action for relief of sore muscles are eucalyptus, cajuput and arnica.

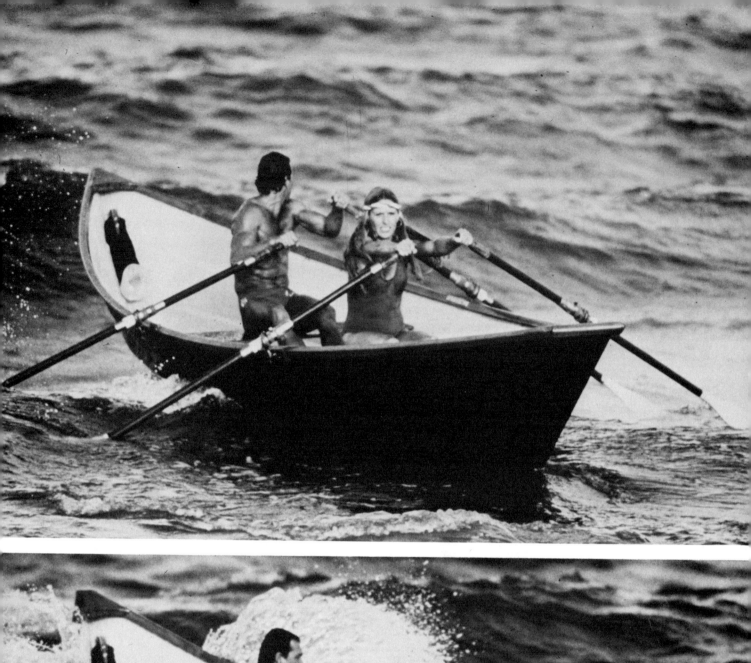

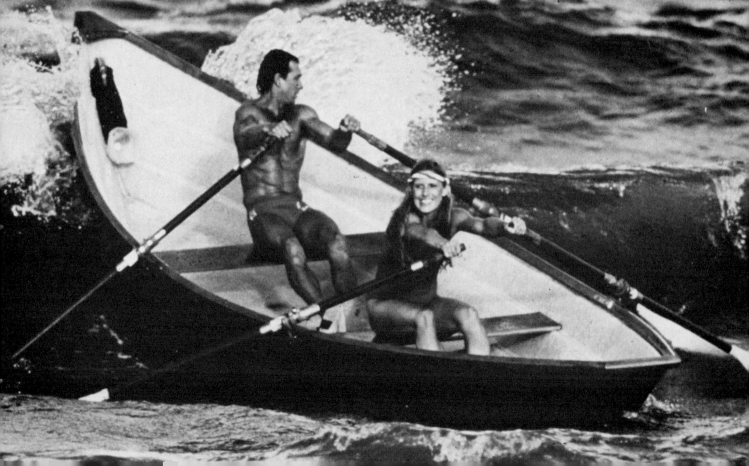

RECIPES FOR STAYING IN SHAPE

LOSING WEIGHT PAINLESSLY

When you're hungry, eat. When you're not hungry, don't eat. This is the key to eating less, which is a foolproof weight-loss technique.

When people ask me how to lose weight, I tell them to eat less, but most people don't realize just how much they really do eat.

The best way to find out in a hurry is simply to write it down. Get a small 49¢ notebook. Keep it with you day and night and write down everything that goes into your mouth. Take a bite out of your friend's sandwich? Write it down. Eat five grapes out of the refrigerator? Write it down. One note—don't cheat on this list because it's just for you.

When you look at it and see what you have actually eaten each day, you'll be surprised. One way to understand how much you eat is to actually see it in writing. Then you can cut out the obvious bad stuff that you ate when you were bored, depressed or whatever. You know what this is better than anyone else.

It's easy to think that just because you eat it fast, and nobody sees you, that it doesn't count. Writing down the list of food makes you accountable to yourself. If you want to actually count the calories, buy yourself one of those dime-store pocket calorie counters and do it. This will reveal even more to you about how good or bad your eating habits are.

Navigating rough tropical conditions with the master, Erik Jersted

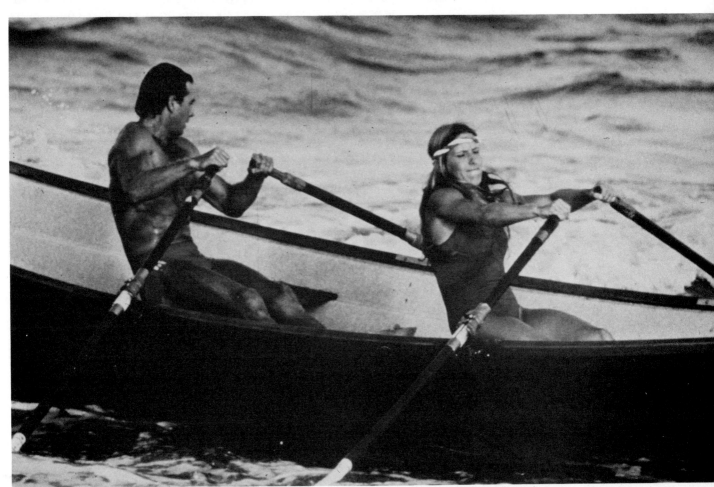

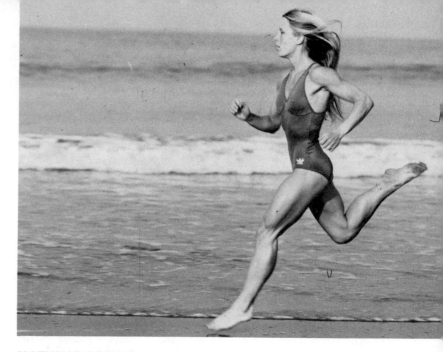

NATURAL FOODS

When you are eating junk food, you have to eat more calories than is necessary to be satisfied. Because the junk food is essentially empty of nutrients, your body's appetite control mechanism (called the appestat) does not signal that hunger is satisfied until a large quantity and number of calories have been consumed. Your body knows when it is being nourished (or not) and therefore says "keep on eating" until there is a sufficient supply of food nutrients.

For instance, I've known people who could put away a whole loaf of white bread at one sitting, but when they eat two slices of home-baked whole wheat or dark rye bread, they're full. The difference here is possibly 1,500 calories for the white bread and 200 calories for the whole grain bread.

The following recipes are made from whole, natural, unrefined foods. The main dishes supply the body with the three essential food elements: protein, fat and carbohydrates. If you use the philosophy of eating "real" foods when you're hungry, then your big surprise will soon be that you don't have to diet. You will be living the eating plan you need.

Fad diets last only as long as the fad, and fast food is the way to get fat fastest.

Eating whole foods like the ones in these recipes will keep you slender and fit easily into your life if you can make this your motto:

When you're hungry, eat.
When you're not hungry, don't eat.

In the meantime, enjoy your food, and bon appetit!

BELIEVE IT

- If you have to ask how many calories it has, you can't afford it.
- Never food-shop when you're hungry.
- Never eat stand-up meals in front of the refrigerator.
- Nobody said you have to swallow it.

SUPERSTAR THIN TIPS

- Avoid salt—it makes you carry water weight.
- Eat slowly.
- Don't keep it in the house and you won't eat it.
- Act like you're already thin—if you've got it, you might just as well flaunt it—stand up straight—pull in your stomach.
- Buy smaller packages of the stuff you are addicted to—you'll save money too—money you can spend on your new thin wardrobe.
- Give away your "fat clothes" as soon as they start growing baggy —your closet will be thinner for it, and you won't have them around to get used to again in the unlikely event that you start to slide.
- Don't skip meals—it only makes you grouchy and you'll over-compensate at the next meal.
- Don't expect to "oink out."
- Boredom is a main cause of overeating. Key on non-food activities to release that depression or anger—sex, for instance, it even burns calories—what a bargain!

DON'T BELIEVE IT FOR A SECOND!

- Chocolate is only bad for people with acne.
- Eating after midnight helps you sleep.
- Cheesecake is just packed with vitamins.
- Dessert helps settle a heavy meal.
- If you eat it real fast, and nobody sees you—it doesn't count.
- Chocolate bars are chock-full of milk protein and energy.
- Ice cream sundaes will calm your nerves.
- It's not me—the scale must be broken.

SUBSTITUTES

For a thin, healthy body, use these delicious, easily available substitutes for common fattening foods.
- For sesame seeds—use poppy seeds
- For salt—substitute dulse or kelp
- For bread, 100 cal/slice—substitute rice crackers, 25 cal/slice
- For cheese—substitute tofu or cottage cheese
- For commercial salad dressing—substitute olive oil and lime juice

HERBS FOR HEALTH

Cooking is really anything you do to prepare food for eating—making a salad or blending fruit for a smoothie. In this section there are tips on how to cook things in ways that can help ease muscle aches and pains, stimulate sluggish systems, and actually increase stamina and endurance.

When using the herbs for recipes, please don't use the bottled, overpriced kind that you buy in a supermarket. They're usually stale. For the best medicinal results and the tastiest foods, grow your own plants in little pots on your windowsill or buy them in bulk at your local natural food store or local ethnic bakeries and delicatessens such as Greek, Italian or Lebanese.

Then buy a mortar and pestle and grind them yourself in your own kitchen. This is easy to do. Just crumple the leaves of, for instance, the basil plant into the mortar, and grind away. It only takes a few seconds and it's lots of fun. The whole production takes no more effort than twisting a pepper mill a few times. Incidentally, you can use your familiar table pepper mill for grinding perhaps less familiar things such as coriander and other such seeds.

GRANDMA'S KITCHEN

My grandmother's kitchen. The bread is baking. The soup is simmering, sending off a wonderful garlic aroma. The room is warm and inviting.

After a thirty-mile run—long hours on a cold road—you enter her kitchen, and the rich warm feeling there seems to heal the tiredness immediately. Someone ought to market "Essence of Baked Bread." I think it's the sweetest perfume in the whole world.

Yet it's not just the warmth and aroma of my grandmother's kitchen that seems so healing. It's the special alchemy of being in a place where the food is prepared with love. It's as if the food takes on the special energy of those kind hands preparing food.

You can tell a lot about people by the way they cook. For instance, uninspired, lobotomized cooking—throwing frozen TV dinners into the microwave night after night—says something about people who don't care or respect themselves enough to feed themselves better food.

IS IT TRUE WHAT THEY SAY ABOUT GINSENG?

It is precisely because of its reputation as an aphrodisiac that I had never tried ginseng. As a very healthy and fit woman in her mid-twenties, aphrodisiacs were certainly not on the top of my list of priorities.

Yet in studying the potent herbs of the world, my readings revealed more and more research on this gnarled little root called ginseng that has scientists buzzing over its possible pharmacological value as an adaptogen, an ergogenic aid, an antioxidant and a life-span extender. Modern science is just discovering ginseng. The Chinese, with their penchant for venerating traditional wisdom, have been using ginseng for thousands of years.

The toxicity test for any substance called the LD_{50} is what scientists use to determine the dosage that will kill 50 percent of the animals taking in that substance. Almost everything has an LD_{50}, even water and oxygen. In one test I read, control animals not receiving ginseng lived an average of 800 days less than the ones who did take it. The moral of the story seems to be that the search for the lethal dose of ginseng ended up extending the lives of the experimental animals.

Ginseng is a remarkable plant that takes six years to reach maturity and unceasing agricultural attention. It is therefore the most expensive popular herb on the market today, with prices ranging from twenty cents a stick for ginseng chewing gum to several hundred dollars for a Manchurian wild root.

Good ginseng products are expensive, but you get what you pay for. Korea leads the world in production of *panax* ginseng, the Asiatic type which is considered by elitists to be superior to the North American *Panax quinquefolium* type because of soil and climatic differences.

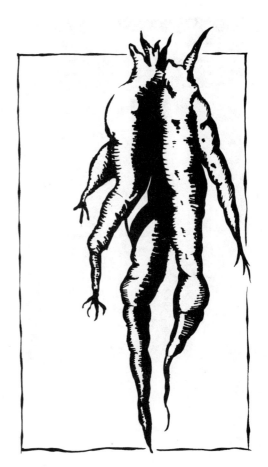

The current North American affinity for things Chinese is seeing the marketing of ginseng products such as chewing gum, lozenges, soft drinks with fizz and hair tonics. My friend Ralph even makes ginseng cookies for his girl friend. At twenty dollars an ounce, though, I'll take it straight in a tea cup with hot water, thanks.

Russian athletes and cosmonauts are rumored to be taking ginseng daily, and this information alone is usually enough to cause North American athletes to swallow the stuff by the gallon. There is no one food substance, herbal or otherwise, that is going to make you run faster, jump higher or throw farther. However, if a plant such as ginseng can supply micronutrients and enzymes necessary to help your body prepare for, recover from and endure the rigorous training necessary for maximum performance, then I feel it's worth going for it! Ginseng is used in so many different ways that it was called a "panacea," hence the botanical name *panax*.

Oh, and in answer to the inevitable question: "Is ginseng an aphrodisiac?" Most scientific research says no. But please don't tell that to Ralph.

BAY LEAVES

My traveling days in Europe often led me to interesting discoveries of plants and natural remedies as local folk and gypsies in different countries befriended me and shared their herbal remedies.

A tour of the ancient marble statues in Rome caused me to notice that athletes in these and other statuary are often holding a sprig of laurel to denote honor, or distinguish the victors of athletic contests.

To this day, laurel wreaths are awarded to the victors of the Boston Marathon and other prestigious races. Its value in ancient times as a revered and powerful herb is almost forgotten now, but the powerful effect of laurel, or bay, leaves, is no less potent today than it was thousands of years ago.

Bay leaves are soothing to the stomach and a wonderful general tonic to the system. They are also an effective carminative. So even though the healing properties of this small shrub may have been forgotten, the leaves of this Mediterranean plant will always be a special symbol for athletes around the world.

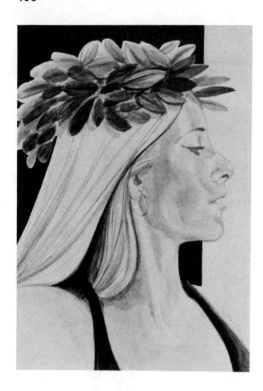

Resting-on-Your-Laurels Tomato Sauce

If you can learn to master this simple tomato sauce, you will have the basis for many a tasty dish from pasta to pizza, and you will indeed have acquired adequate laurels to rest on. Diluted with vegetable stock, it makes a wonderfully light bouillon base that can be eaten alone as an appetizer to a main course, or as a base to a hearty soup. Chilled, it becomes a unique and zesty alternative to dead, canned tomato juice. Either way, do not use aluminum utensils when making tomato dishes—or any dishes for that matter—as the acid in the tomatoes will pit the aluminum, resulting in a bitter metallic taste to the dish, which is not only unpleasant but poisonous.

And while you have the bay leaves out, you may wish to make a note of the fact that women in the Mediterranean countries have always made an effective remedy for colicky babies by boiling water with several bay leaves in it, cooling it, then pouring it into the baby bottle. Works great for grown-ups too—the bottle is optional, of course.

20 plum tomatoes	1–3 bay leaves
1–3 cloves garlic	2–4 tbsp olive oil
3–5 leaves fresh basil (or 1 heaping tsp dry basil)	

Peel tomatoes by scalding them briefly in boiling water so the skins come off easily. Peel cloves of garlic and put them in a blender with a small piece of the skinned tomato. Blend for 2 seconds. Add the rest of the tomatoes to the garlic mixture in the blender and give it a quick whirl of 2 to 3 seconds. Remove from blender and put mixture in a pot. Bring it to a simmer, *uncovered.* Chop fresh basil (or measure dry basil) and add it and the bay leaves to the sauce. Simmer until it reaches the consistency you like (I prefer to bring it just to a boil, but judge for yourself). It doesn't need to simmer long—approximately 5 minutes—unless you aren't using plum tomatoes. The others are more watery. Add raw, cold-pressed olive oil (available in any natural food store) just before serving.

Remove the bay leaves before serving—they're impossible to chew. Rest on your laurels and bon appetit!

Feeds: as a spaghetti sauce, two athletes or four regular guests.

Superstar Tip: A bay leaf placed in the containers you use to store grains and oats will keep out the mealy bugs (the ones that *look* like sesame seeds.)

Vina's Potato Pizza

At one point in my life, I carried only two telephone numbers in my wallet in case of emergency—my lawyer's and the pizzeria's.

Pizza was a powerful addiction to overcome in subsequent years of food reform, yet I still submit to it in New York City, where Vina D'Agostino, an accomplished Italian gourmet chef, never fails to delight me with this original recipe.

3 lbs potatoes

2 eggs

2 tbsp fresh parsley (or 1 tbsp dry)

2 tbsp olive oil or butter

1 lb mozzarella cheese

1 tsp oregano

Resting on Your Laurels tomato sauce to taste (see p. 108).

Scrub potatoes with a veggie brush. Quarter and drop them in boiling water—just enough to barely cover. After cooking, discard water and mash.

In a separate bowl, beat two eggs with parsley. Add to potatoes with olive oil and mix well.

Spread potato mixture on lightly oiled pizza pan very thinly, pressing with palms of hands to one-half-inch thickness.

Bake in a hot oven (400°F) until golden brown.

Slice or shred fresh mozzarella to desired taste onto crust. Add tomato sauce and re-insert in oven for five minutes. Then remove, and put remaining mozzarella on top. Shut off oven and re-insert to melt cheese. Sprinkle oregano lightly, and serve.

Feeds: two pizza addicts—four athletes—six polite guests.

GARLIC

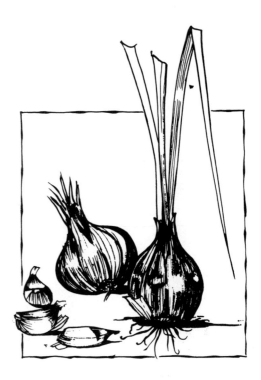

It may be my gypsy blood, but of all the herbs, I think garlic is the most magical.

Cleopatra gave her lovers meals heavily laced with garlic in order to increase their stamina. Aristophanes believed that garlic could restore a man's virility. Hercules always carried garlic and admitted it to be his source of power. In Egypt, garlic was given to the slaves in a ration so that they could endure the hard labor of building the pyramids. Pliny wrote that "garlic acts as an aphrodisiac beaten up with fresh coriander and taken in pure wine." The Greeks used it in ancient times as a poison antidote, and Europeans in the Middle Ages fought the plague with garlic potions.

Folk remedies throughout history are full of references to garlic, and it has been taken to cure ills such as bronchitis, asthma, dysentery, tuberculosis, poisoning and impotence. It's only recently that scientists have begun investigations of this little bulb with so many powers. In the 1940's, allicin, a sulphur compound, was isolated from garlic in an American experiment. Subsequent research has found garlic to be very high in the trace minerals germanium and selenium, adding anticarcinogenic qualities to the long list of ever-growing claims. My grandmother credits garlic with lowering her blood pressure after doctors told her that death was imminent because of her life-threatening high blood pressure.

Skeptics of garlic are always quick to point to the long and extremely diverse list of human complaints in which garlic has been claimed as the cure. Some of the claims *do* seem extravagant, but then nature has some powerful remedies.

In the years to come, researchers and medical experts will continue to probe the pungent cloves of this little plant, and the new information will certainly be welcome.

But I'm not waiting for the verdict to come in. Garlic is a great taste for dozens of dishes. If you've never tried it, don't knock it. After all, could Cleopatra, Hercules and my grandmother all be wrong?

Sensational Zucchini Sauce with Garlic

This is a green sauce with garlic used in the way you would a tomato sauce—very good on noodles or as a sauce for all the grains, rice, millet or bulgur, for instance. It's also a good companion to potatoes—baked, boiled or mashed. I've used it on sandwiches which need a sauce to keep them from being dry. Enjoy.

2 medium zucchini squash
2 bay leaves
1¼ oz pine (pignolia) nuts, shelled
2 cloves garlic

4 fresh large basil leaves (or 1 tbsp dry)
⅛–¼ cup olive oil (according to taste)

Cut zucchini lengthwise in quarters, then cut in half. Bring 1 inch of water with bay leaves to a rapid boil in a one-quart saucepan. Add zucchini and boil for 3 minutes.

Remove and discard bay leaves. Add remaining ingredients and put everything in blender and blend well.

Note: When keeping this sauce warm, do *not* keep on direct flame. Use a double boiler only, as actually *cooking* the sauce on a flame can make it taste bitter.

Feeds: four athletes—6–8 regular guests. Serve on top of noodles. Chop ½ cup of fresh parsley and sprinkle on top—eat heartily.

CAYENNE

My old friend Tony, now 75, first introduced me to cayenne pepper by way of an old country remedy called *nastoika.* A handful of the pepper pods are steeped in a bottle of vodka. A one-shot glassful was given to me after I had finished a grueling cross-country ski race, complete with frost bite and hypothermia (the opposite of heat stroke). After one swallow, my lips, mouth and throat were aflame. My eyes were watering and I felt that further irreparable damage was imminent. Within moments though, the fire subsided. My shaking from the cold had stopped. My blue fingernails and lips were pink again due to the restored circulation, and I felt positively glowing.

Years later, on a carpentry job, I learned of cayenne's styptic qualities when Tony sprinkled some cayenne powder on a deep cut. The burn was incredible! But the bleeding stopped in seconds, a scab formed, and I didn't need stitches. There was no infection later.

Cayenne is used in herbal formulas for high blood pressure, anemia, colds, flu, skin disorders and heart ailments. North American Indians valued it as a systemic immunizer (to ward off disease), and in the West Indies it is used to reduce fevers. In Morocco, I saw people fumigate their apartments by burning cayenne pepper on a low flame, sealing off the room, and then returning after the smoke and the bugs had cleared.

Cayenne pepper is probably valued most, however, as a stimulant of the energy and functional ability of the body. Therefore, it has great potential for us as we strive for maximum performance.

Keep in mind when cooking that cayenne should be added last, as heat lessens the potency of the herb. Also, be sure to accustom yourself gradually to the fiery power of this herb, and you will know another of nature's tremendous endowments.

Blazing Lentils with Cayenne

You're in charge of adding the cayenne.

2 cups lentils (dry)
6 cups water
2 cups chopped celery and
    leaves
1 cup diced carrots

4 bay leaves
4 potatoes, diced
    dash of cumin
½ cup fresh parsley
    cayenne to taste
1 medium onion, diced

I prepare this by putting all the ingredients in a crock pot, and leaving it to simmer at a very low heat all day while I'm out. Then, I add cayenne and it's ready for the evening meal. The fast method is to boil at a high heat for one hour after having soaked the lentils (overnight) previously.

Feeds: four athletes as a main dish, or six regular guests.

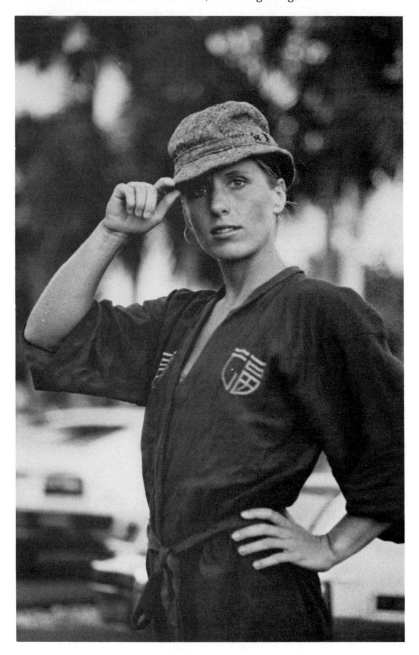

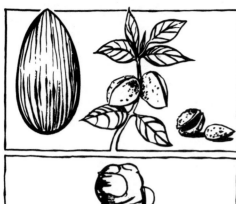

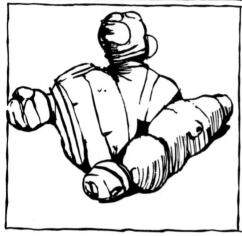

MILLET

Ginger was brought to the New World by the Spanish conquistadores and it was established as a major crop in the West Indies in the sixteenth century. The islands are still the Western World's largest suppliers of ginger, an herb popular today in both medicinal and culinary circles.

A long run on a cold road is enough of an occasion to prompt me into making this millet dish with ginger in the starring role. Ginger enhances circulation to cold areas of the body, where muscle tension can restrict blood flow. The warming qualities of ginger are the most esteemed by its fans. Internally, ginger's effects in increasing circulation can relieve cramped muscles, stiff joints and cold extremities. Digestion is also enhanced by ginger, and as a hot tea, it is used to relieve menstrual cramping and headaches.

I have often appreciated ginger's ability to banish sore throats caused by breathing, dry cold air. Externally applied, it will act as a rubefacient, promoting circulation in a specific area.

Millet is a complex carbohydrate of the type that is essential for replacing muscle gylcogen after a long endurance workout.

Ginger's effect on the body is stimulating, and its effect on this millet is unusual and delicious. I hope you agree. Bon appetit!

Mighty Millet for One with Ginger

½ cup millet	1–2 tbsp butter
2 cups water	40 almonds
1 piece fresh ginger root	¼ cup finely chopped fresh
½ the size of your thumb	parsley
1 tbsp lemon juice	

Put millet and water in a pot and bring to a boil, thereafter reducing to a medium-high flame 15 to 20 minutes, until done and water is absorbed.

Grate ginger root and stir into millet with lemon juice and butter.

The almonds may be roasted lightly for 3 minutes under the broiler if preferred for taste. The almonds and parsley can be stirred into the millet, reserving some for the top as a garnish. Serve in a bowl, and eat with a spoon. Add a salad and you have a hearty meal high in protein and complex carbohydrates.

Feeds: one hungry athlete.

CHIA SEEDS*

Chia is related to the sage family, and the tiny seeds were once the staple of the Indian diet in Mexico and the southern United States. It was considered to be a cereal, and was cultivated the way corn was.

Chia seeds are an energy and endurance food used by the Indians for centuries. Rommel's troops used chia seeds in their forced marches across North Africa. I routinely sprinkle them on salads and soups. A little goes a long way, as chia seeds expand to 8 to 10 times their original size when combined with water.

* Chia seeds and any other unfamiliar ingredients in this section are obtainable at your local natural foods store. If they are temporarily out of stock, ask them to order it for you.

Creamy Chia Seed Dressing

1 tsp chia seeds	2 tbsp honey
1 tsp paprika	1 tsp marjoram
1 clove of garlic (or more to taste)	16 oz of plain yogurt
	1 dash tamari sauce
2 tbsp lemon or lime juice	½ tsp smoked nutritional yeast

Mix all ingredients well and chill overnight. Add water if necessary to achieve desired consistency. Thick, I like it on baked potatoes. Thinner, I use it on salads or as a dip.

Supreme Sprout Salad

1 cup sunflower sprouts	1 cup lentil sprouts
1 cup alfalfa sprouts	1 cup grated beet or carrot

Toss together or arrange in separate mounds on a dish. Grate the beets or carrots and either create another mound in the middle of the dish or sprinkle on top. Reserve a few sprouts of alfalfa for a garnish. Use chia dressing.

Feeds: two.

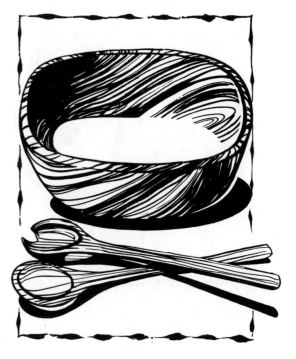

LEMON AND SAGE

Lemon juice is one of nature's strongest antiseptics, and sage is certainly one of the world's most versatile herbs. It is a tonic and purifier of the liver and kidneys according to the old writings, and was greatly respected for its calming effect on nerves and muscles, John Wesley being one of sage's more articulate spokesmen on the topic. He claimed the use of sage tea as the answer to palsy. The American Indians of the desert venerated sage as a sacred herb capable of increasing the life span.

Theophrastus, Pliny and Hippocrates have all written of its herbal powers, and once again our modern civilization is discovering that nature is still our greatest apothecary.

Naked Dressing

Your salad need never go naked once you have mastered this simple dressing. The secret to its flavor is in preparing it well beforehand so that the oils and juices can meld.

⅝ cup olive oil	2 tsp Italian herbs or ½ tsp each of oregano, sage, basil and thyme
¼ cup lemon juice	
⅓ cup apple cider vinegar	
1 clove of garlic, pressed	

Tabouli Salad

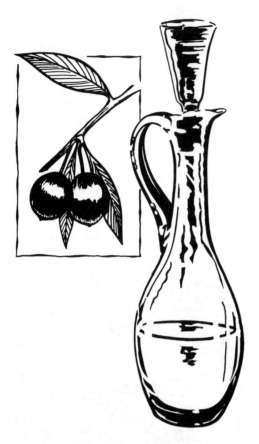

This recipe comes from the Middle East—lands that conjure up visions of perfumed gardens and fountains in palace courtyards of former sultans. Tabouli salad is one of many eastern dishes perfumed with herbs—in this case, mint.

Mint is a digestive and has been used since ancient times to calm the nervous and muscular systems. Mint refreshes and soothes. In this recipe it's the ingredient that makes the dish a standout. The bulgur (cracked wheat) is an excellent complex carbohydrate source for refueling muscle glycogen that is lost in demanding workouts. You can make the tabouli in the morning, and then keep it chilled until after your evening workout. If this is my plan, I prefer to add the tomatoes just before serving. Eat as is or with pita (pocket) bread and sprouts. And may your dreams that night be of starry Mediterranean skies.

1 cup bulgur (cracked wheat), fine	½ bunch mint
1 bunch scallions, finely chopped	4 medium tomatoes
	4 lemons juiced
2 bunches of parsley	¼–½ cup olive oil
	tamari sauce to taste

Soak bulgur in water for a few minutes. Squeeze dry by pressing between palms of hands. Chop scallions, parsley, mint and tomatoes very fine. Add bulgur, lemon juice, olive oil and tamari sauce. Mix well. Serve with lettuce leaves and sprouts.

Feeds: three athletes—6 polite guests.

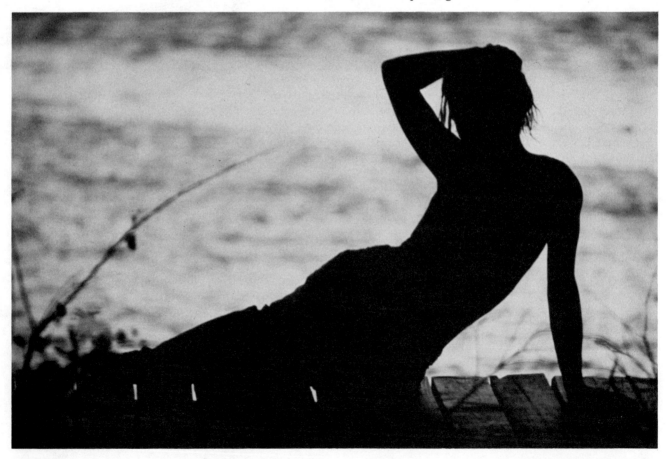

Victory Salad

This salad was first served to my dinner guests not as a main dish. However, after finishing the last bite of my salad, I looked up to see three pairs of hungry eyes gazing at me intently. Finally, someone said, "Gee, I'd sure like to just have more of this for dinner." Everyone quickly agreed, so I went back to the kitchen, did the whole thing over again, and returned to serve the same salad once more. It was devoured, and I ate with them, feeling very proud indeed to have made my dinner guests so happy. The dinner had been to celebrate a marathon win that day, but I felt my real victory at that moment was in pleasing my dining companions. I hope your guests enjoy it as much as we did.

THE CAST

Celery: So revered by the Greeks that it was given as a prize to the Olympic winners in ancient times. It is high in electrolyte minerals, and the Greeks esteemed it for its rejuvenation qualities.

Parsley: Rich in manganese and iron. It's a good natural diuretic and stimulant. When eaten with garlic, takes the odor from the breath. As an herb it's also used for thyroid deficiencies, diabetes and genito-urinary tract infections.

Oregano: Helps digestion and is soothing to the stomach.

Basil: For circulation and also useful for curing catarrh (congestion). A stimulant.

---

1 bunch celery
3 cucumbers
1 lb fresh mushrooms
6 oz green large olives (drained weight)
1 large bouquet of fresh parsley
   juice of 1 lemon
4–6 tbsp olive oil

2 cloves crushed garlic
3 tbsp dulse flakes or 3 tsp kelp
1 lb tofu cubed in 1 inch sq or ¾ lb of unsalted swiss lorraine cheese,* cubed
1 tbsp dried oregano
1 tbsp dried basil

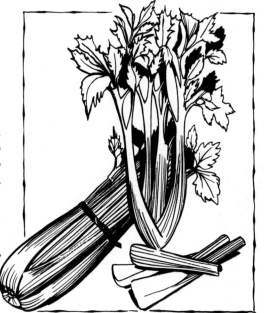

Slice celery diagonally in ½ inch pieces. Peel and slice cucumbers in half lengthwise, then in chunks. Wash mushrooms and chop into halves. Cut olives into pieces and discard pits. Chop parsley, not too finely. Combine in large salad bowl, and add remaining ingredients. Toss thoroughly and serve.

Feeds: two athletes—or four regular people.

* Swiss Lorraine cheese may be purchased 90 percent salt- and fat-free at specialty stores.

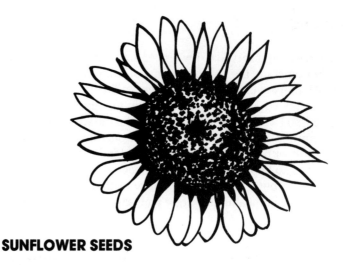

SUNFLOWER SEEDS

As soon as the head is formed on a sunflower plant, it always faces the sun, turning its head from east to west each day to absorb life-giving rays of sunshine. It is a remarkable plant—very easy to grow, hardy, resistant to disease and never needs poisons sprayed on it for bugs.

The seeds are loaded with B vitamins, and the oil is very rich in Vitamin A for strong eye health and beautiful skin. The seeds have tremendous quantities of minerals, especially phosphorous, calcium and zinc. In the Ukraine, where men carry sunflower seeds in their pockets to eat as snacks, the incidence of prostate problems is very low, due no doubt to the Vitamin A, Vitamin E and zinc content of the seeds. The sunflower is the national emblem of the Ukraine, and while I'm not sure if that's the only reason why, it seems like they're definitely on to something. Try planting some seeds in your garden this summer—the bright sunny flowers can grow over six feet high, and you will be rewarded for growing them with an abundance of seeds to eat.

Macho Salad with Sunflower Seeds

You don't have to be macho to enjoy this salad.

3   medium carrots   ⅔ cup raisins
    (approximately 1½ cups   ½ cup sunflower seeds
    grated)

Mix ingredients, garnish with parsley and serve with yogurt honey dressing.

Feeds: one athlete as a main dish, or two people as a side dish.

Yogurt Honey Dressing

1 cup yogurt
1 tbsp lemon
1 tbsp honey

Beat well. Delicious on Macho Salad or fruit salad.

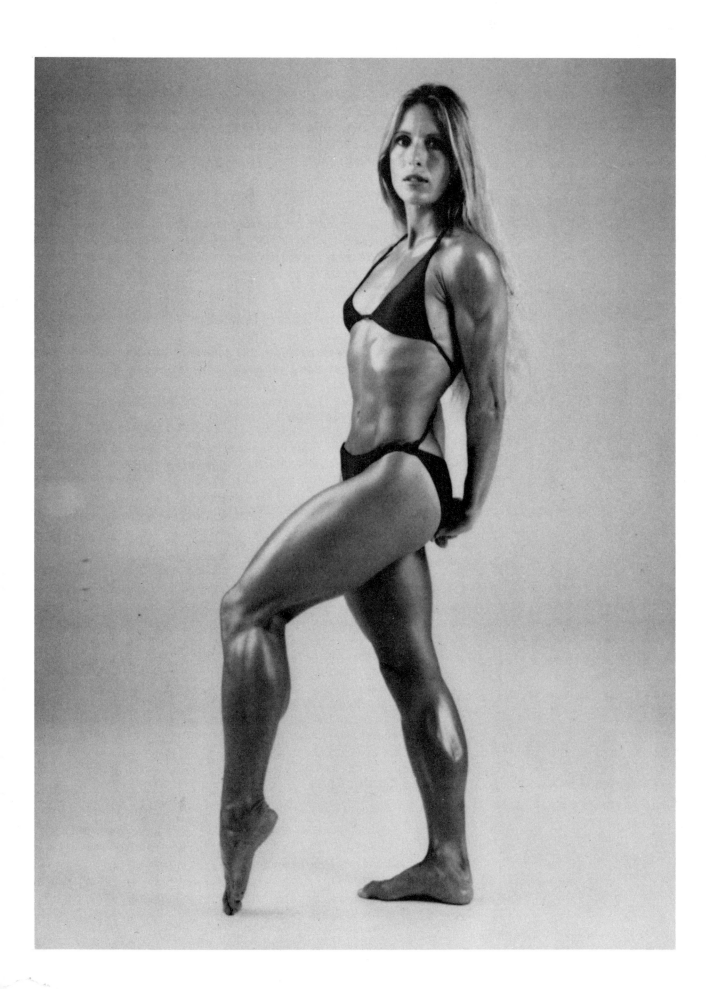

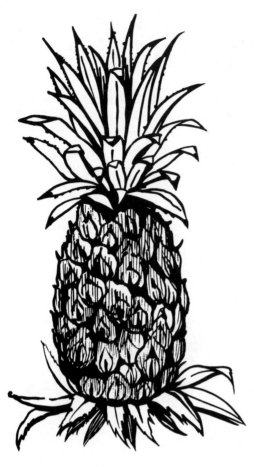

PINEAPPLE AND STRAWBERRY

Pineapple is loaded with bromelain, a proteolytic enzyme which has the ability to eat away dead tissue in the body. It is therefore a useful food for athletes, to be eaten when an injured part is swollen and the swelling must be reduced. Ice, of course, is the immediate external first aid treatment. The captain of my "pit crew," Dr. Jack Kahn, first introduced me to this pineapple treatment after having great success with it in treating pro-football players' post-game swollen knees.

When lactic acid building in my muscles causes soreness, I also find that eating a whole fresh pineapple helps to flush the lactic acid out, and aids in repairing the tiny tears and strains that hard training and racing can produce.

Pineapple Strawberry Morsels

Cut pineapple as shown. Mix in fresh strawberries and, if desired, serve with yogurt honey dressing.

Pineapple/Cranberry Cocktail

Blend equal parts of pineapple and cranberry juice and serve chilled over ice. A delightful thirst quencher.

Prune Whip with Cinnamon

Cinnamon is soothing to the intestinal tract, and is used in many countries as a natural antibiotic and stimulant.

2 cups prunes	cinnamon to taste
1¼ cups apple juice	1 banana
¼ cup almonds	

Soak prunes overnight in apple juice. Remove the pits, and with the remaining liquid throw in blender. Add nuts, cinnamon and banana, and blend to a purée. Serve chilled in a wine goblet with a sprinkle of cinnamon on top and garnish with a single almond. *Note:* Unsulphured prunes vary in dryness, so extra apple juice may be needed in order to blenderize smoothly.   Feeds: four.

Fig Confections

8 oz. dried Calymyrna Figs (or 1 dozen figs)	½ cup shredded coconut
¾ cup finely chopped walnuts (or almonds)	2 tbsp carob powder
	½ tsp cinnamon
	3 tbsp honey

Snip stems from figs. Set aside. In a bowl, toss together nuts, coconut, carob and cinnamon. Drizzle honey over mixture. Mix and knead with hands until it sticks together in one big lump.

Using the handle of a small spoon, poke a hole in the blossom end of the figs and form a cavity. Stuff with mixture, making a mound on top of the inside of fig. Chill or freeze. Makes one dozen stuffed figs.

PAPAYA

Papaya is often called the king of fruit because of its cleansing, purifying and vitality-inducing qualities.

Papaya contains papain, a vegetable pepsin that can dissolve several hundred times its own weight in protein. In Africa, I've seen women smear milky papaya leaf juice on their meat before cooking in order to tenderize it. Another tenderizing method used by native people in the tropics is the practice of wrapping their meat in papaya leaves and keeping it this way overnight.

Living in the tropics for many years myself, I've enjoyed the succulent delight of the papaya just as they come—right off the tree. The seeds are very easy to grow, only you must plant enough to be sure of a male and female tree growing together. The male tree bears only flowers, and the female only fruit.

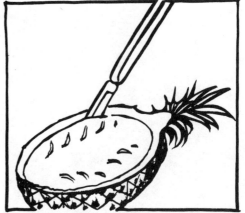

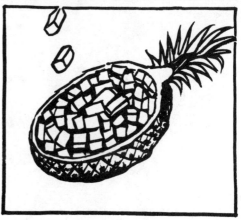

Papaya Fruit Salad

1 papaya
1 banana
1 cup strawberries

Feeds: one athlete or two as a side dish.

Papaya Smoothie

1 cup plain yogurt
1 papaya
1 banana

1 cup strawberries
2 drops vanilla (or honey)

Put yogurt in blender, then add the other ingredients slowly with blades turning. A few drops of vanilla extract and honey to taste may be added if desired. The best result is achieved if all the ingredients have been refrigerated before using.

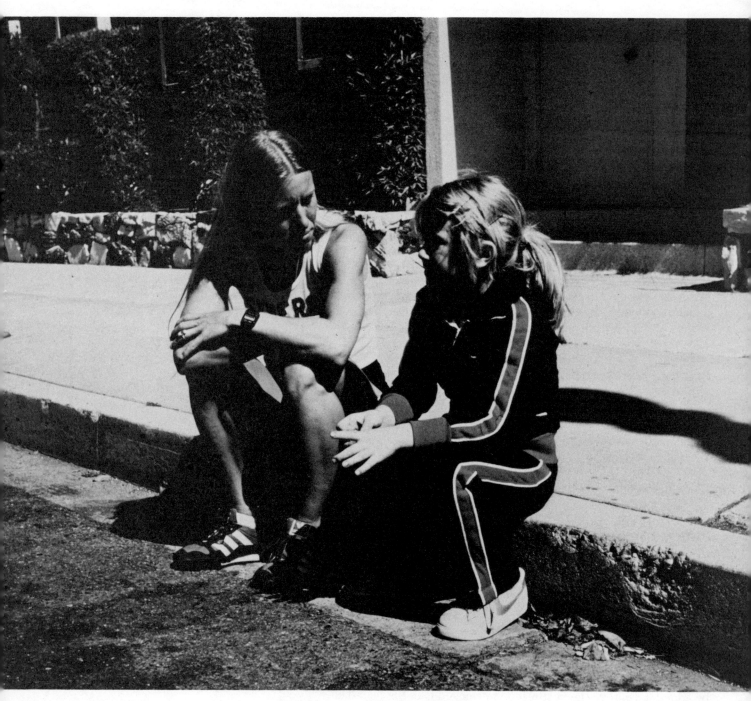

Comparing notes with a future Olympian

5
QUESTIONS AND ANSWERS

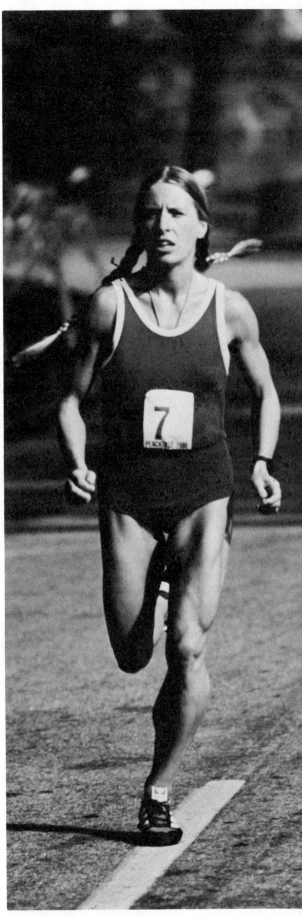

People stop me on the street, in supermarkets, restaurants and even airports to ask me how to get fit, what to eat, and how to be healthy. At my own lectures around the world, executives, homemakers, children and even elite athletes always have question after question for me on their personal health programs. And each day my mailbox at the office is stuffed with envelopes containing letters from dear people from Saudi Arabia to the South Seas. The kindness of people everywhere with their constant hope and encouragement for me has touched me many times, and this book was actually begun in response to this communication. Those who write to me are under seven and sometimes over seventy. The common thread is that they are always looking for a way to improve themselves. To become healthy and to continue their commitment to *getting stronger.*

The following questions are on the most-asked topics. The answers are as complete as I can give you without getting extremely technical and perhaps obscuring the issues with too much information.

I'm reminded of a story in which a seven-year-old boy runs to his parents and asks, "What's sex?" The parents, being modern, garden variety conscientious types, instantly trundle out a few encyclopedias and a stack of color posters and diagrams. After a long, complicated philosophic and physiological explanation, the young boy's face drops, and the parents nervously ask him what's the matter. "Oh, nothing," replies the boy, "Only how am I going to fit all that on this I.D. card, where it says *sex:*?" I hope my answers are closer to the mark.

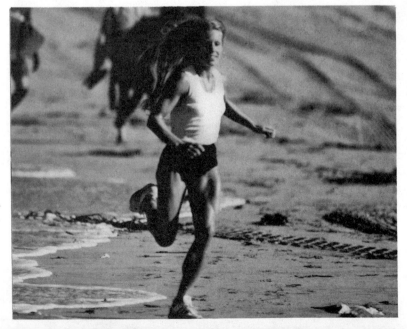

Peach Tree Road Race, 1980

121

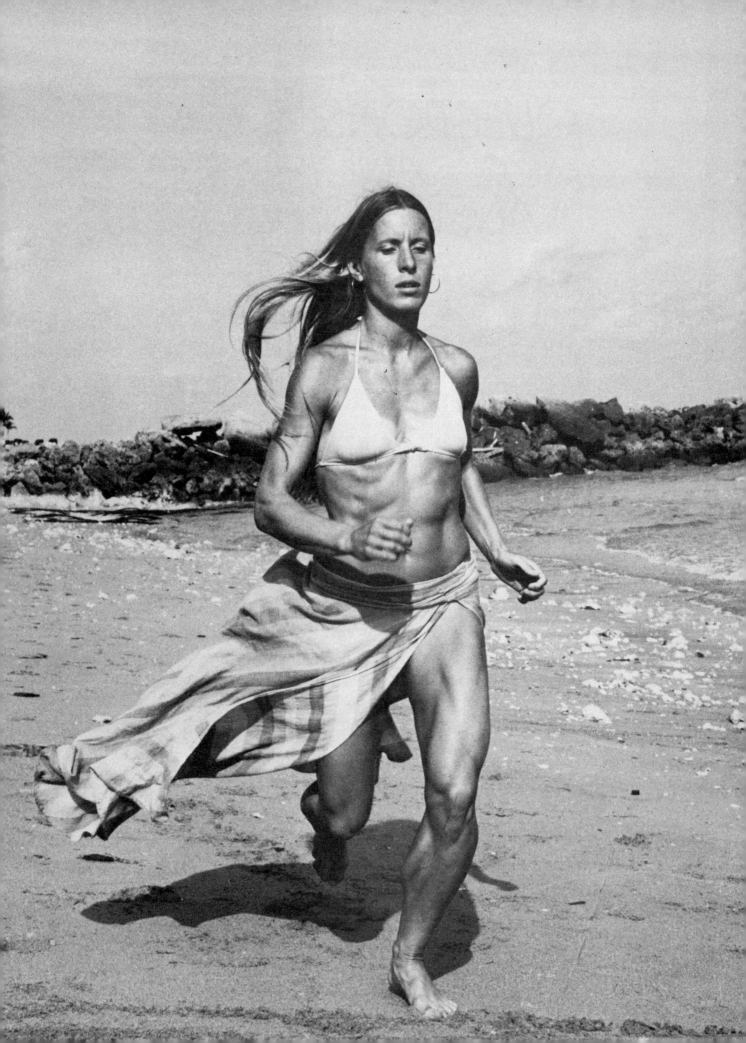

RUNNING

Q. Should I wear a bra when I run?

A. Yes. Not only does it support but it also helps to prevent a common problem with runners—chafed nipples. What happens is that your nipples become cold and erect while you're running, and if your shirt is nylon, which is particularly irritating, or mesh, the constant rubbing against the unprotected nipples causes chafing. This is a problem faced by men as well, and if you prefer to run without a bra you can borrow one of the solutions offered them: place adhesive strips over the nipples or cover them with Vaseline.

Q. Should you have sex before a competitive sport?

A. Medical studies have shown that sex depletes men of Vitamin E and therefore does affect their athletic performance. Women, on the other hand, do not lose Vitamin E, but most women athletes will tell you that the myth about sex before sports is true. It does take away your aggressive edge.

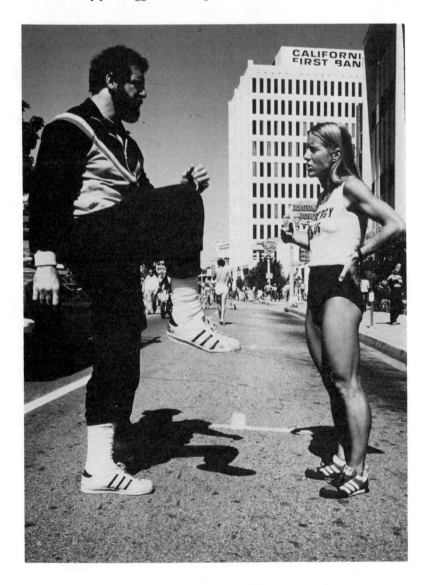

Pro-football superstar Lyle Alzado and I discussing speed drills

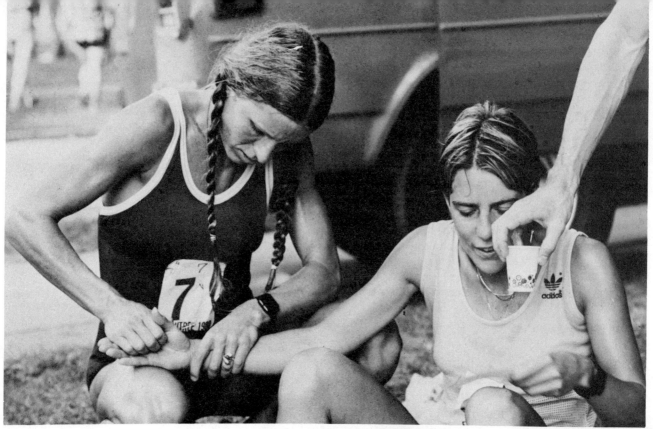

With Kitty Consolo, relieving pain with acupressure after a grueling race

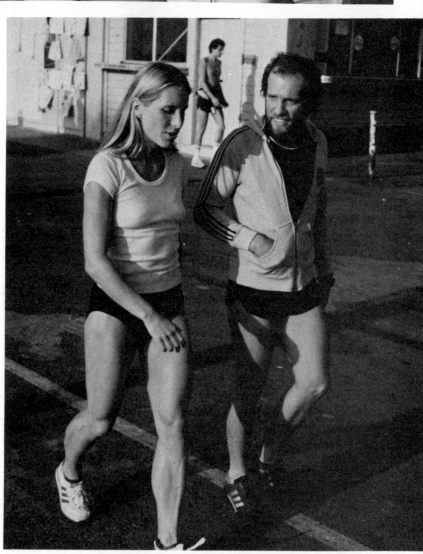

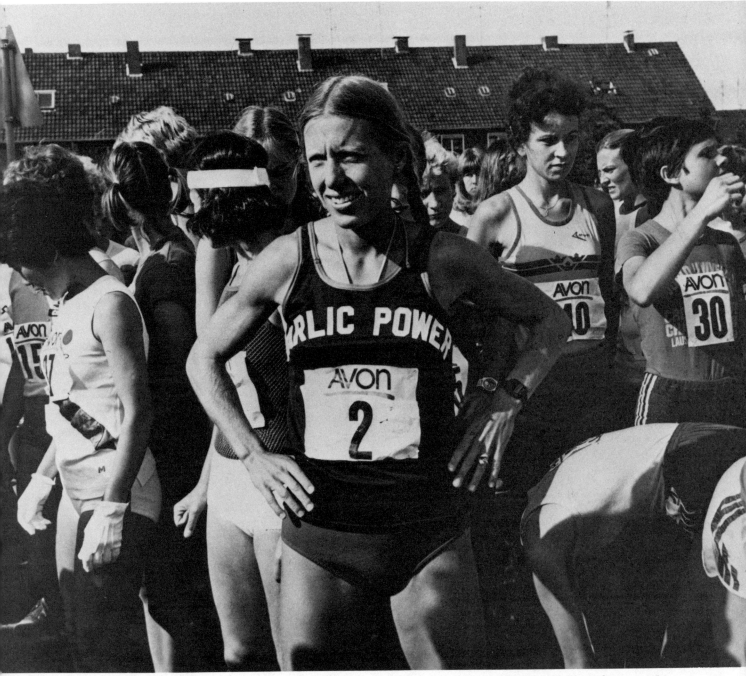

The starting line—the World Championships, West Germany, 1979

Q. Is there really such a thing as "runner's high"?

A. Yes. The "runner's high" is a natural high you can achieve while exercising, because hormones called endorphins are released from the cortex of the brain. Endorphins are chemically one link away from morphine and are known to relieve depression, increase sense of well being and decrease pain, which is why they are known as the "morphine within." Unlike morphine, however, endorphins are not habit forming.

Q. Should I eat before running?

A. No. You shouldn't eat for at least two hours before strenuous exercise in order to avoid stomach cramps.

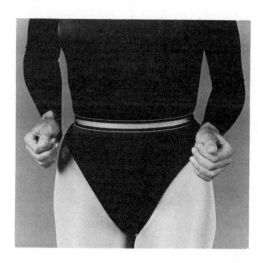

Q. How do you hold your hands when running?

A. Your thumbs should rest lightly on the first crease of the index finger. The pressure used would be enough to hold a strand of hair in place. The thumbs should also point forward.

Q. Do you feel that weight lifting helps running?

A. Sure does. Strength + Flexibility = Speed.

At the starting line of my first marathon, one of the men I was standing beside looked at my arms and said, "You'd better stand at the back of the pack. You're too big to finish a marathon." He was in shock at twenty-three miles when I passed him, but in marathon tradition cheered me on. Later, he asked me about a lifting program.

Lifting makes you stronger. You look better, you feel better, you run faster and you have fewer injuries. I was ostracized for years by some of my competitors because I looked so much different than they did, but lately I've read that even some of them have incorporated some weight training into their regimes. I chuckle when I read interviews where some of my former critics now extol the virtues of weight training. As I've said for years, it works.

Winning the NBC Peacock Run, 1980

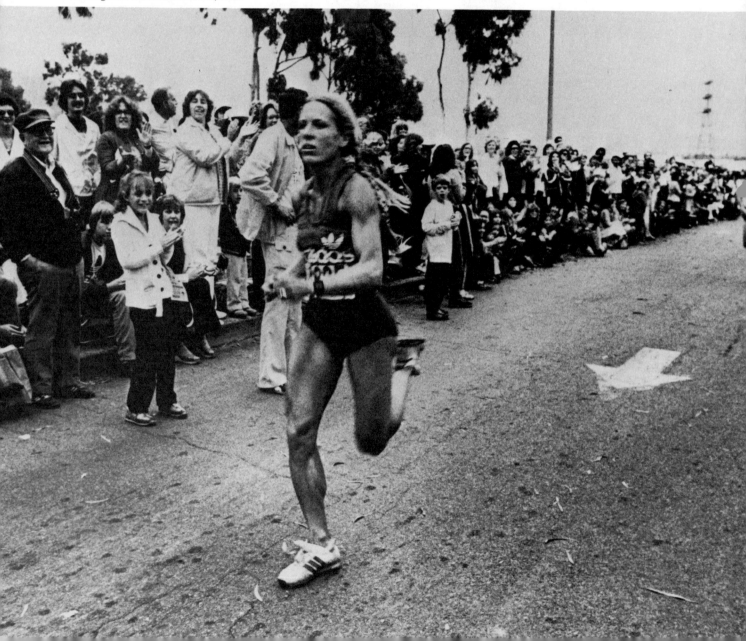

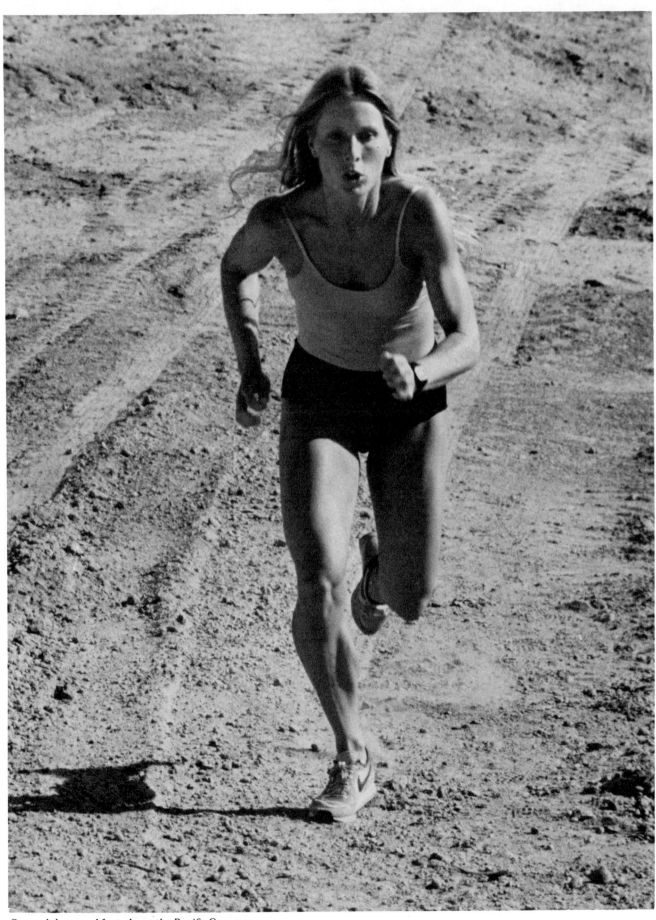

Several thousand feet above the Pacific Ocean
in the Santa Monica Mountains

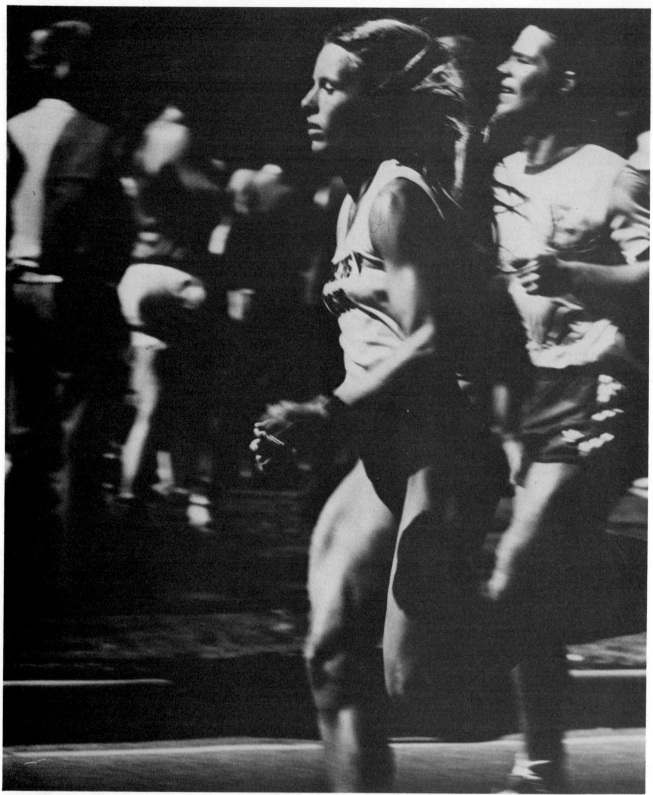

Winning the Brentwood 10-K, 1980

Q. What about arms?

A. Your arms are more important to your speed than most people give them credit. Avoid holding them close to your chest, or poking your elbows out to the side. Hold your arms at approximately a ninety-degree angle from the elbow and allow them to swing back from the shoulder—*straight back.* Practice in front of a mirror, or facing a friend who can help correct you. If you find this ninety-degree angle tiring, then read over the arm exercises and then *do them!*

Q. What do you do for "stitches"?

A. Those pains in your belly right next to your ribs that you get when
exercising sometimes can be attributed to a number of causes:
1. Weak stomach muscles.
2 Undigested food or gas in the intestines.
3. Drinking very cold water when you're hot and sweaty.
4. All of the above.
5. None of the above—add your own.
During one marathon, I developed stitches near the eleven-mile
mark. I was leading the race, but with those stitches, how to continue? Hearing once that sit-ups helped, I lay down in the middle
of the road, and banged out forty sit-ups right there on the hot
sticky pavement. Another runner, who had been trailing me,
caught up, and said, "If you think I'm going to do sit-ups on top of
this, I quit!" (And he did.) Fortunately, the stitches disappeared
and I continued on to win.

However, I have since found a better cure for stitches that is
less disruptive for you (and your fellow competitors):
A. Blow all the air in your lungs *out* while pushing your abdomen
   out.
B. Now, without breathing, suck your abdomen in.
C. Repeat several times.

This creates a vacuum pressure that eases gas and cramps.
Eventually, you will be able to do this while exercising, without
ever stopping. It also strengthens your stomach muscles and aids
in elimination—try it first thing in the morning.

Actually, it's the same principle used in belly dancing—that's
where I learned it. So even if you never get a "stitch," you can learn
this exercise, get a ruby for your navel, and be a hit at your next
party.

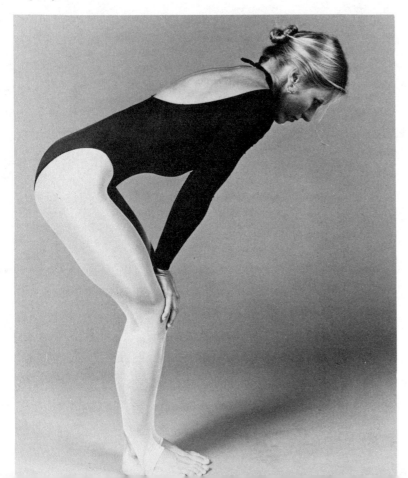

Q. Do you feel you have a limit to how fast you can run? And with the women's world record in the marathon coming down every year, do you think that women will reach their limit soon?

A. It's been said that you only use 10 percent of your brain, and your brain controls your body. When one person breaks a world record, for instance, the limit is re-set, and then everybody starts running that time. If I have a limit to how fast I can run, I have yet to find it, but perhaps this search for it is what fuels me.

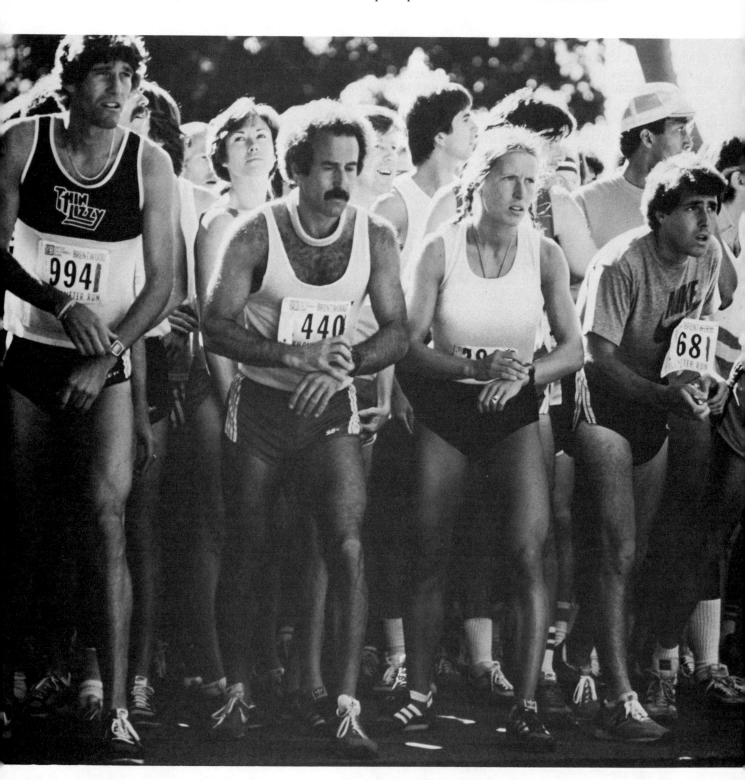

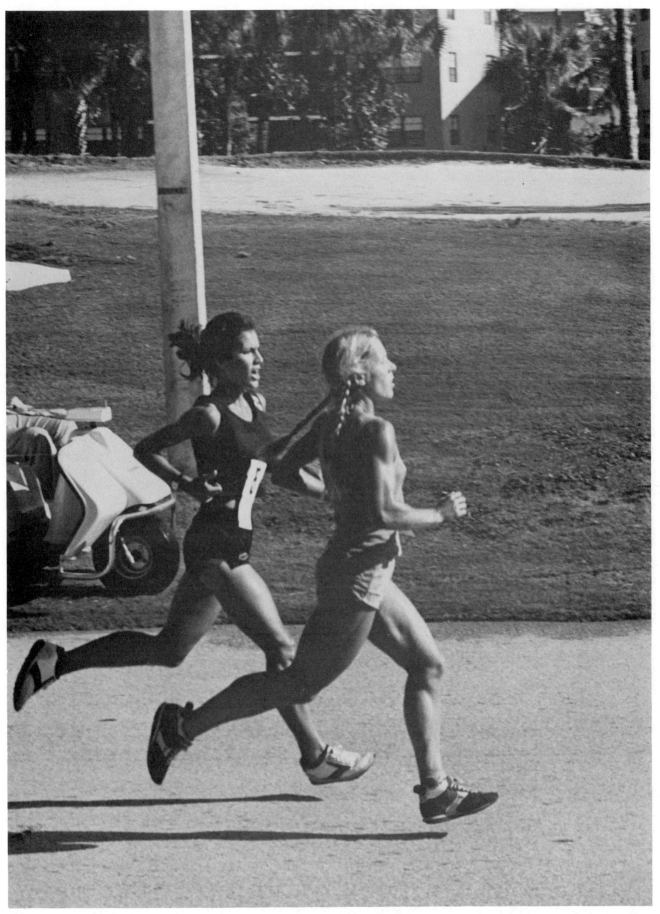

*Pushing the pace with Gayle Barron in the
Avon Regional Championships*

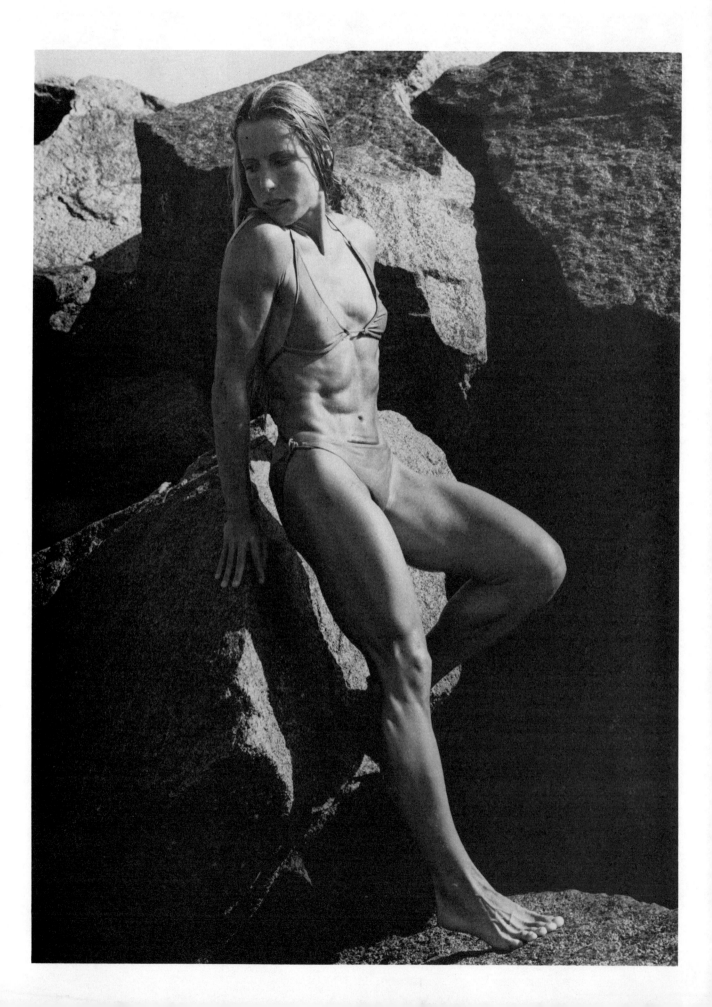

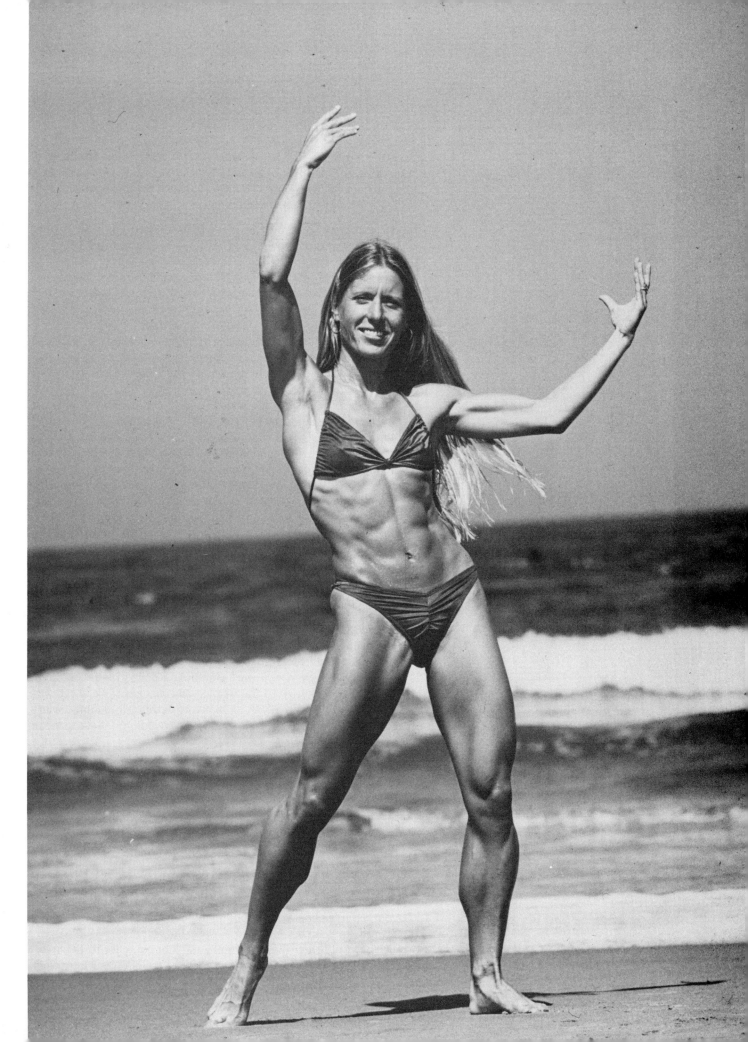

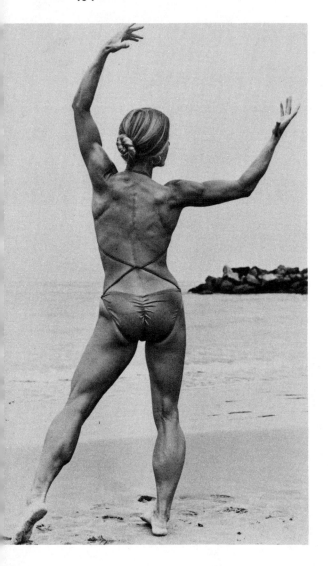

THE MIND

Q. I've tried them all—I start with good intentions on my diet and exercise program, and then it only lasts for about two weeks and I gain back all the weight and more, because I get depressed. I don't know why. I just seem to lose interest and get bored with it all.

A. Turn to page 23, "Thirteen Ways to Make Sure You Don't Go for It," and copy them down.

We all temporarily lose interest in a project at some point. Try and figure out why *you* do. Are you in the "afraid to give it your best shot so that you'll always have a good excuse" category? Are you using food and inertia to act out boredom, or dissatisfaction with some other part of your life? For example: "I feel rotten—I'm depressed that my boyfriend/girl friend never called me, and I just ate a whole bag of chocolate cookies so I'm off my program. I might just as well forget the whole thing, and start again next Monday."

First of all, your plan should only be as strict as your heart and head can stand, and still retain the joy of living. Are you setting impossible goals? (Review "Commandment for Success No. 1.") Be realistic. Are you expecting your whole life to become perfect immediately because after years of neglect you finally decided to get yourself into shape? Again, be realistic. Deciding to go for it will give you rewards right away, but it's the *accumulative* effect of the commitment over time that has the biggest impact. Remember, even Rome wasn't built in two weeks, and neither is your life.

Next, stop buying the food that you know is junk, and if it's not around the house, you won't eat it when the phone doesn't ring, or you feel lonely, bored, or depressed or whatever it is that sets you off.

Another important fact to keep in mind is that just because you've binged out once after you've started, that is *not* the signal to bail out altogether. Accept the fact that you are human and then get back on the track.

For instance, if you were watching a tennis match, and one tennis player conceded the whole game because one serve was fumbled, you'd probably think that very extreme and unnecessary behavior, right? After all, one fumbled serve does not have to mean a forfeit of the whole game.

It's the same with having one binge-out or missed day of exercise. Realize that you made a mistake, and then go for it. And don't wait until next Monday to do it.

Another few words on putting off the completion of your plans. Is it a way of providing some negative stimulation for yourself by sneaking that Danish or skipping your workout? This could be an ancient response to situations we once knew as kids—ducking gym class or snitching candy from the jar. It may have been heart-pounding way back then, but surely there are better ways to get some excitement now. After all, you're only cheating yourself now. For heart-pounding enjoyment, let's not ignore the rewards of good sex—it even *burns* calories.

Also, consider the pattern of your "not going for it" behavior. Do you corner friends and co-workers to confide your latest fail-

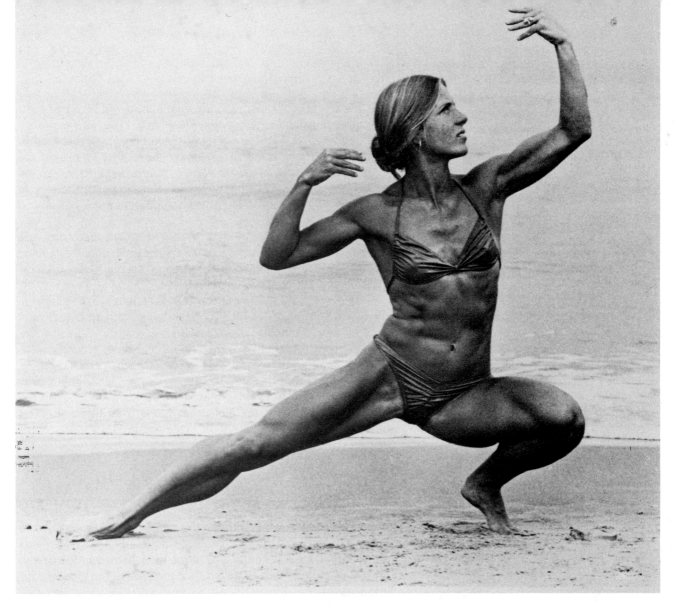

ure? Or are you silently defying your conscience, stubbornly chiding yourself but not doing anything about it either? Are you into it even more deeply, blaming everyone around you for your own failure to get it together, and therefore having a built-in excuse? (Review "Commandment for Success No. 6.")

Whatever your reasons or whatever the pattern of your procrastination, applying "Commandment for Success No. 7, Don't Get In Your Own Way," is particularly appropriate, as are the following:

1. List your reasons for not going for it (mentally or actually writing them out). This is the past.

2. The next step is thinking of what you can handle *now,* in the present. For instance, if you haven't done a spot of exercise in ten years, do you feel like you could handle twenty minutes of walking every day before dinner? Then that's what you do.

3. Finally, think of the future. This is a type of immediate gratification reward system. You've punished yourself long enough by procrastinating. *Do it anyway.* You've got excuses and extenuating circumstances not even covered in my answer to you? *Do it anyway,* just for the beauty of it. Going for it has rewards that are limited only by your imagination. Still feel bored being in a brand new get-in-shape program? *Do it anyway.* Being fat can get pretty boring too. I know.

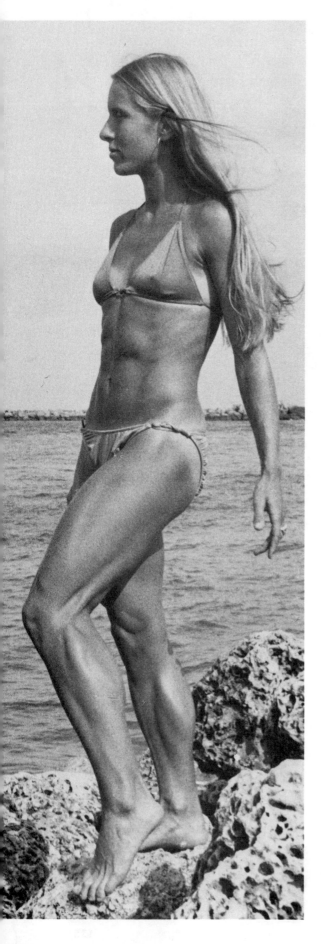

Q. How do you manage stress?

A. Fasting is a great preparation for what I know will be tough business meetings and negotiations. Also, I avoid the business lunch and dinner, as I feel that eating at these times is detrimental to digestion. If these meetings are unavoidable, I try to suggest the restaurant from a list I always carry of natural food places around the country. Then, eat sparingly. Journalists in particular love to interview you over lunch or dinner. I try to steer them instead to a walk by the ocean, for instance.

An answering service is a great investment and saves you from constant interruptions that cause stress. I pull out the phone at bedtime. Nothing worse than someone (usually a race director or journalist) waking you up at midnight.

Being organized is another way to keep things from piling up. I have one day a week which is "Gayle's day" and on that day my management company doesn't schedule any meetings for me. They are very protective of my privacy and time, which is absolutely marvelous for me. And as I travel so much, it eases my mind to know that they are always taking care of business for me. Now that's what I call stress (free) management.

Environmentally, my diet protects me from those stresses, although I'd rather not have to be protected from pollution, which is why I moved from Los Angeles.

Of course, the very best stress management is to be healthy, and be in shape. Then the stress seems to just roll right by you.

Q. I used to be 5'2" and 150 pounds. Now I'm 105 and feeling great since I started jogging and playing racquetball. I would like to know if it's normal to notice men's physiques. When I was fat I was just happy if a man even looked at me twice. Now I suddenly find myself attracted more to the athletic guys. Have the men in your life always been athletes?

A. I've spent fifteen years surrounded by the Olympians, world record holders and great athletes and dancers of the world, and I admit I'm spoiled rotten by seeing the marvelous sculpted bodies of these men every day of my life. Even sexier, though, is the pure energy of their intelligence and supreme motivation to achieve—because to have a great physique without a mind is to be a statue.

It's natural for you to be attracted to the more athletic men now. You've become an achiever, and you want to meet someone who shares your newfound zest for sports. That's understandable. The man in my life has to be athletic. After all, if we're going to run off into the sunset together, I want to be sure he can keep my pace!

Q. It starts about a week before a competiton—I just can't seem to sleep at night, wake up tired, look at my watch every fifteen minutes in the dark. Help! I know my training has been good and I usually win when I get to the competition, but is there anything I can do?

A. If you consume any caffeine at all (tea, coffee, cola, chocolate bars, etc.) now's the time to stop. The excitement leading up to your competition is normal—after all, that's what you train for: to compete. However, your restlessness and insomnia are obviously caused by negative stress. Keep in mind that the tapering of your

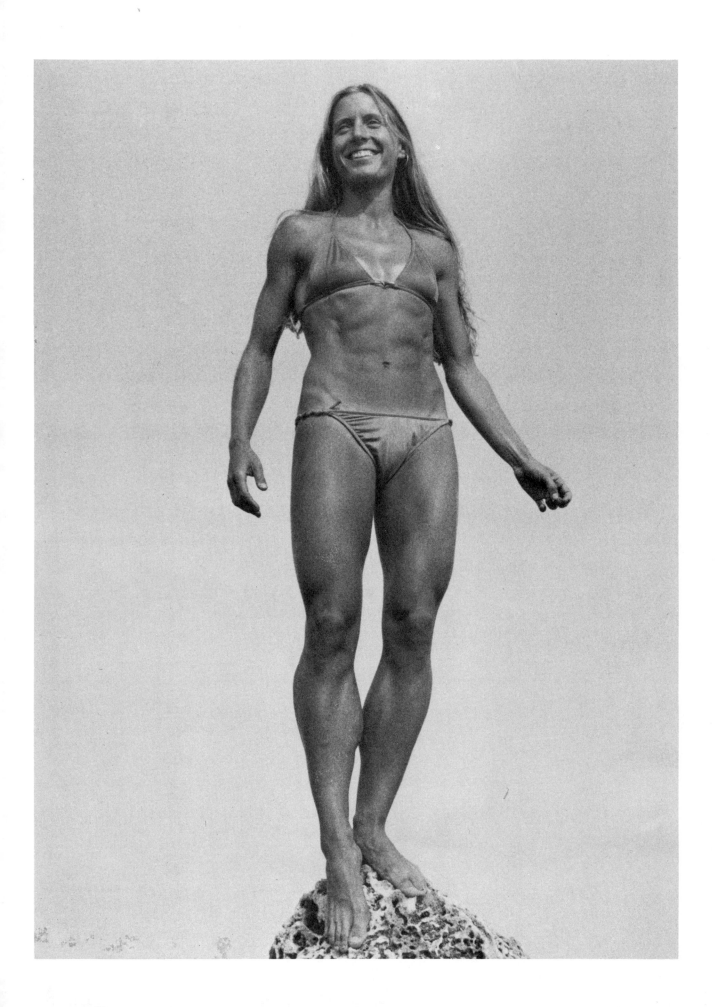

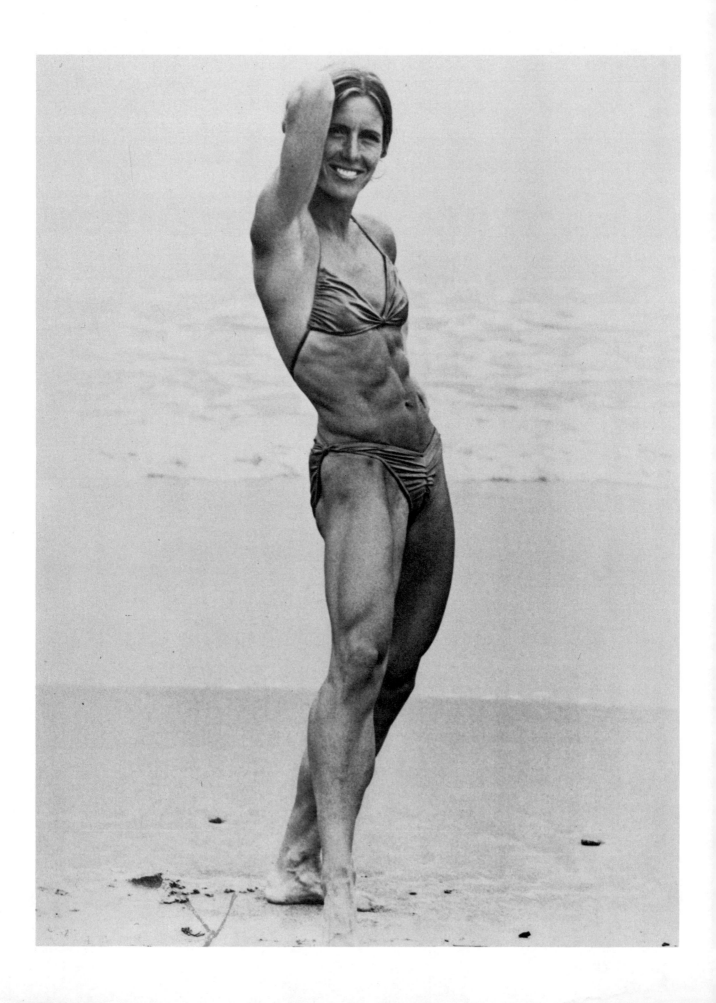

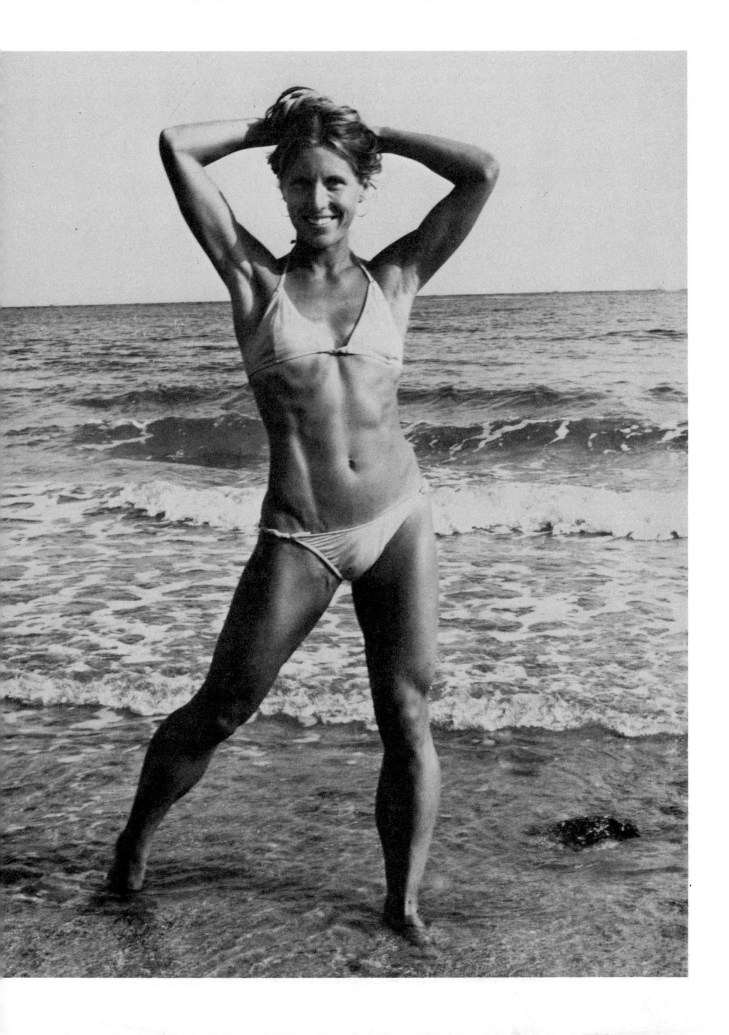

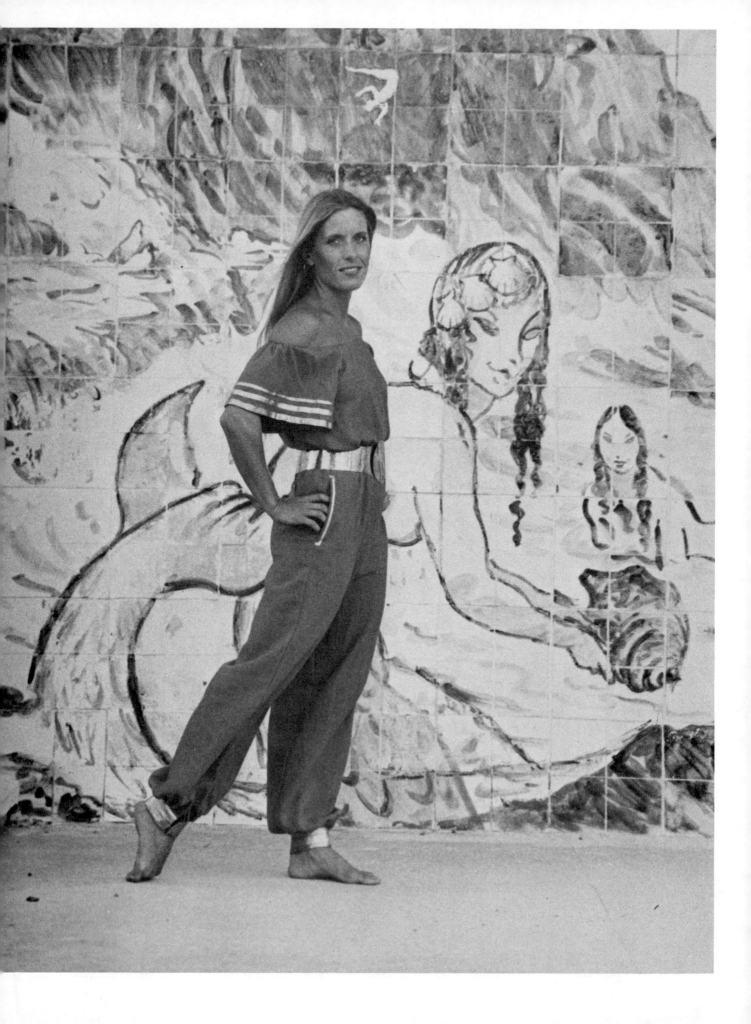

training regime before the big event is releasing an enormous amount of energy that is otherwise spent in sweat. So use it. Go to a movie, or take a walk at night. Various teas have served to calm me during those slow-moving days before the race—including chamomile, mint and valerian root brews. ("Staying with It—Herbal Remedies" list more.)

Are you getting enough calcium? Dolomite tablets will often help here. Tryptophan (an amino acid) is the ingredient of milk that aids in sleep, and is available in tablet form.

Reading a good upbeat novel also calms me sometimes, as do slow dancing, bubble baths and massage (not necessarily in that order). Don't rule out late-night television—now there's a real soporific if ever there was one!

Q. Do you ever wake up in the morning and feel ugly, fat and completely out of shape, even if you felt great the day before?

A. Absolutely. I know the feeling well! I've looked in the mirror on quite a few Monday mornings and winced—and this is after running about thirty miles the day before.

It's unbelievable how bad you can feel on these days—even the most tiny imperfection can make you want to wear a brown paper bag over your head all day.

This is a sign of fatigue, and on these "I feel ugly days" I usually plan something fun for a workout—maybe jumping up and down on a trampoline, rowing in the ocean or running somewhere scenic—like by the ocean, or on a pine needle trail.

For my mental attitude, I schedule a movie or some live music. Buy yourself a new red toothbrush. If your budget allows, treat yourself to that new record album you've wanted, or how about getting a massage?

Whatever you do, don't mope around brooding about the fact that you feel less than perfect. If you're worrying about how you think people see you, remember that not everyone has 20-20 vision.

Q. Do you believe that to be a good athlete you must dedicate every waking moment toward your goal?

A. Athletics is not my whole life. It's a great part of it, but not everything. I feel it's important to love, to create things, to appreciate the art of living as well as what I call the honest working of your muscles.

I've seen many athletes who have spent their whole lives inside a swimming pool, or an ice rink or a gym, and never had any real life experience. The same goes for people I call professional academics. You can be book smart and life stupid. "Street smarts" are valuable, too. I tell the young athletes that I coach—especially those with that indelible imprint of obsession on their souls—that athletics are important, but so is learning truth and finding out what there is to learn.

THE BODY

Q. I'm sixty-five years old. Is it safe for me to start exercising?

A. There is no age restriction on exercise. I've started several people in their eighties on exercise programs, and my own parents, who had never run before, started running at fifty-eight. The only restrictions are those advised by your doctor. No matter what your age, have a physical examination before you begin running; if your blood pressure checks out and your doctor says exercise is indicated, then *Go for It!* I've organized exercise and track clubs for new mothers and their children, and the preschool toddlers outran their mothers because children run all day long. For them, running is play. The same should be true for you.

Q. What is your fitness regime?

A. In addition to running fifteen to thirty miles a day (thirty on weekends only), I also lift weights daily, train with a dancer (he used to dance with Martha Graham), do sit-ups and other calisthenics. All this is daily. Three times a week I swim one to two miles, cycle ten miles on a stationary bicycle, walk up steep hills or mountains (at least 2,000 feet, otherwise it doesn't seem to do that much good). I'm also learning tae-kwan-do. Once every two to three weeks I either race ten or fifteen kilometers or do a time trial.

Q. Is "making weight" bad for you? I wrestle at a class that's now about fourteen pounds *under* what I weigh, and I find it harder and harder to make weight for the competition.

A. Why don't you work out hard, get stronger, and wrestle at the next weight class up? Dropping fourteen pounds every time you wrestle can only dehydrate you dangerously and weaken you for the match. It's also a terrible strain on your entire body. Unless you're carrying fourteen pounds of fat, I advise you to discontinue this practice. And if you are fourteen pounds "overweight," why not keep your goal weight *all* the time by dint of controlled eating and working out?

Q. Will exercise give me big muscles? I'm sixteen and I like sports, but I still want to look feminine and not like the Incredible Hulk or something.

A. First of all, keep in mind that there's only one *man* who can look like Lou Ferrigno, the Incredible Hulk, and that's Lou Ferrigno! Secondly, allow me to say that a woman who develops her muscles through sports will only *accentuate* her body's feminine curves by sculpting a sleek, sinewy body that's taut and muscular in a way that will never be mistaken for a man's.

Judging by my fan mail, the athletic look is *the* look for the woman of the eighties. Muscle is no longer the sole domain of men. Women of today are finally rediscovering what our pioneer grandmothers have known all along about getting stronger. Strength is beauty.

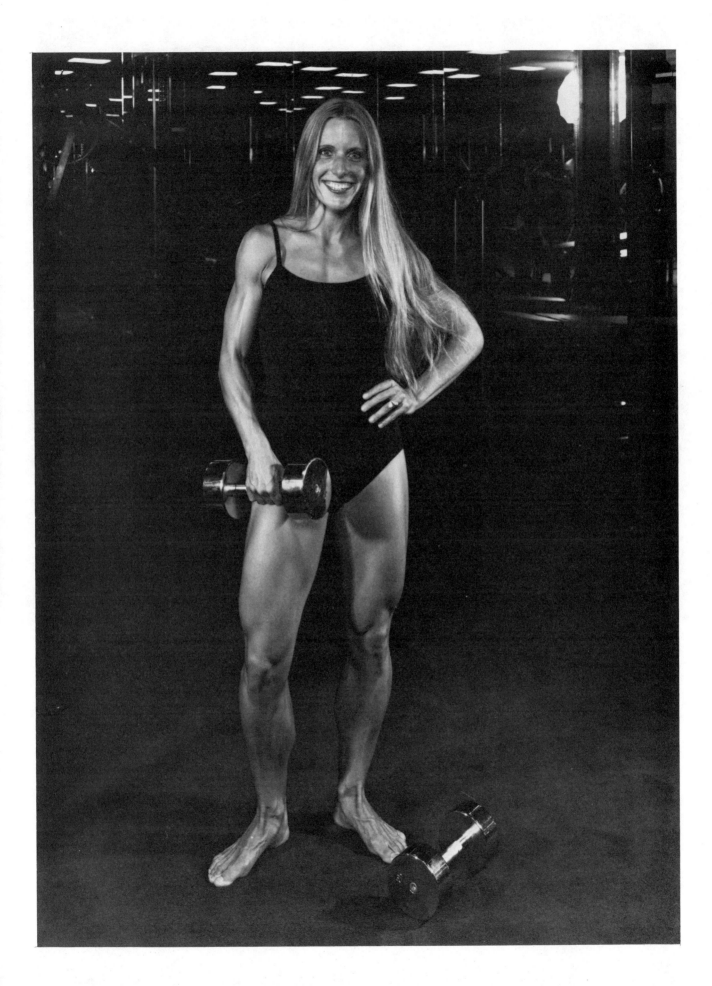

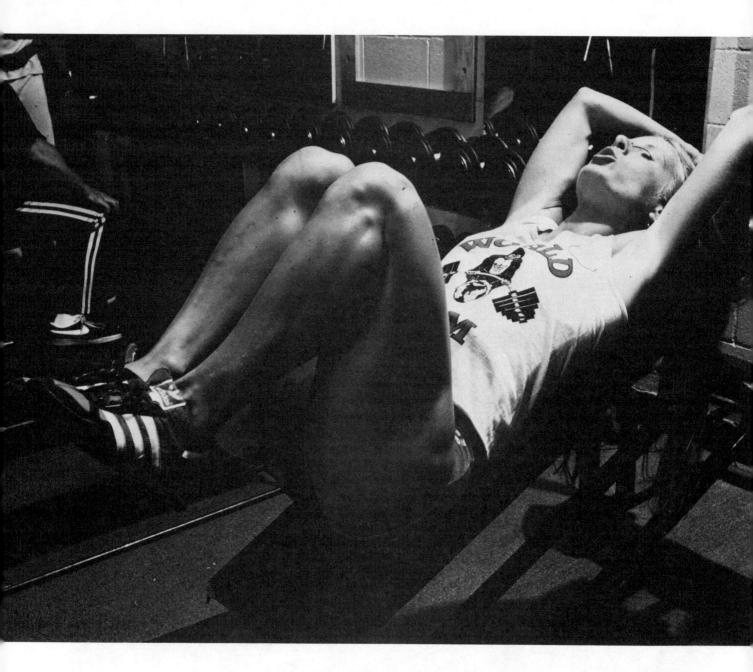

Q. Can you *really* spot reduce with vibrator belts, sauna wraps and rubber sweatsuits? My husband wears one of those thick rubber wrap arounds, and he swears by it, but frankly, I don't see any difference on him. At least at my spa, I figure that the vibrator belt will help me lose a few inches because it's massage. We have a bet on this. Who is right?

A. You're both wrong. There's no such thing as spot reducing. Now you can *firm up* any area by exercise, but those sauna wraps and your husband's rubber wraparound only promote perspiration, and water loss is the only thing you can experience with these. The fat remains to haunt you. And those vibrator belts can do wonders for aching muscles, but the fat they jiggle only gets tickled, and it doesn't fall off you. I'm sorry you both lost the bet, but with the extra time on your hands because of this resolved predicament, take heart. That cloth-backed spongy rubber from your husband's wraparound is the very stuff used in the fanciest of insoles by the running elite. Cut out a pair for each other and have enough left over for a new pair on your birthdays!

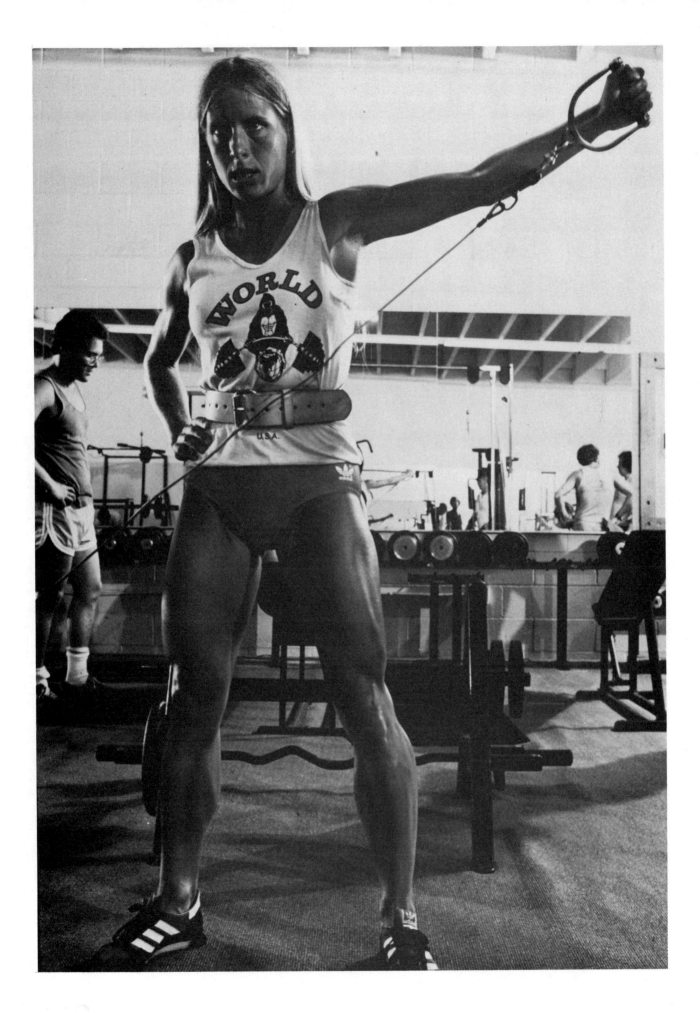

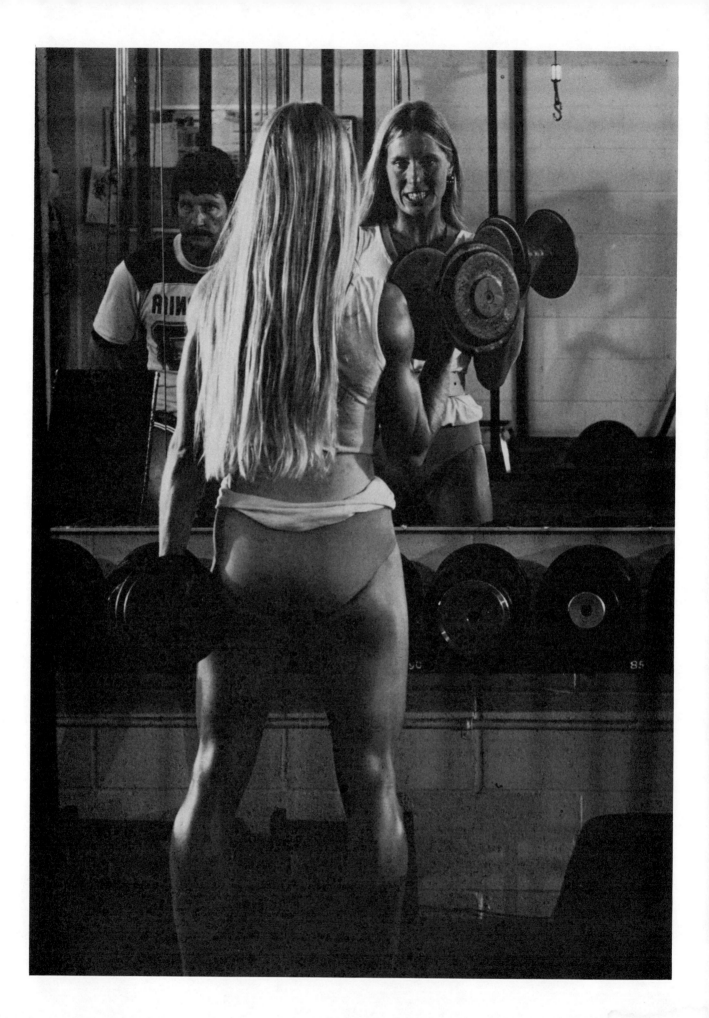

Q. Sometimes I just feel too exhausted to get to sleep after hard training. Is there a cure for this?

A. I know the feeling well. Happily though, there are a few things that can help you.

  The first is to make sure you don't eat a heavy meal at night right before you go to bed. Allow at least two hours between the evening meal and bedtime. Otherwise your body is at work during the "off" evening hours and you even wake up tired. If you feel the need to eat before sleeping, raw carrot and celery juice induces relaxation.

  Herb teas can also have a calming effect on your nervous system (see "Staying with It—Herbal Remedies"). At times the excitement of having done a tough workout will leave you a little frazzled mentally as well as physically. Easy stretching and a hot bath can do wonders as well as a little TLC (tender loving care).

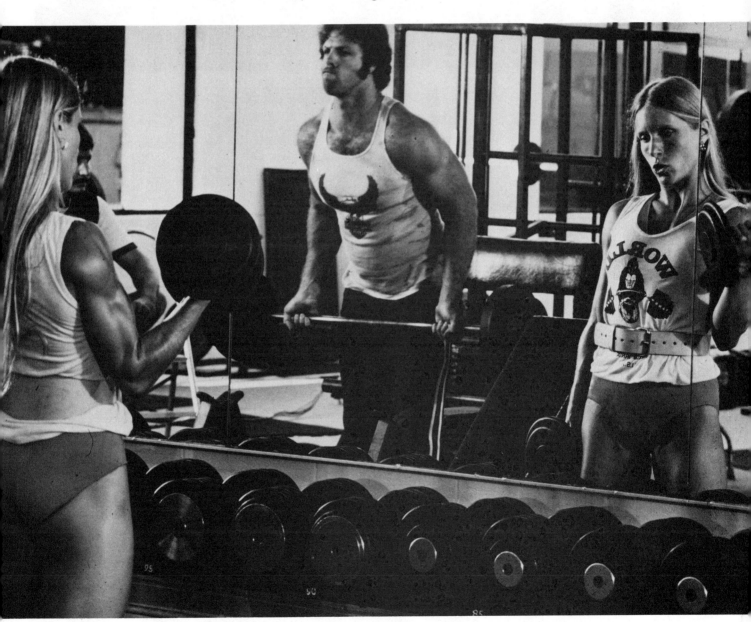

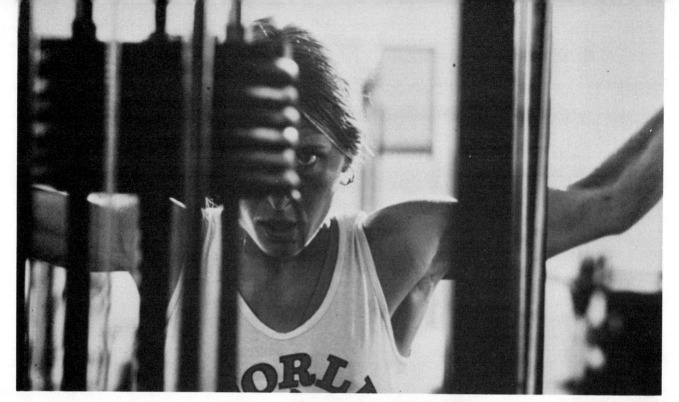

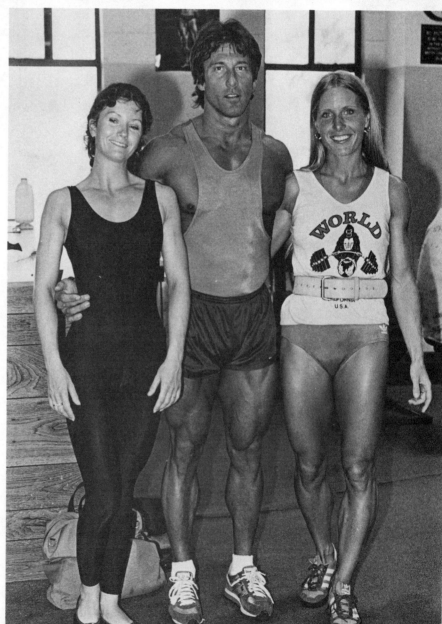

After a hard workout with Mr. Olympia,
Frank Zane, and the French body-
building champion in California

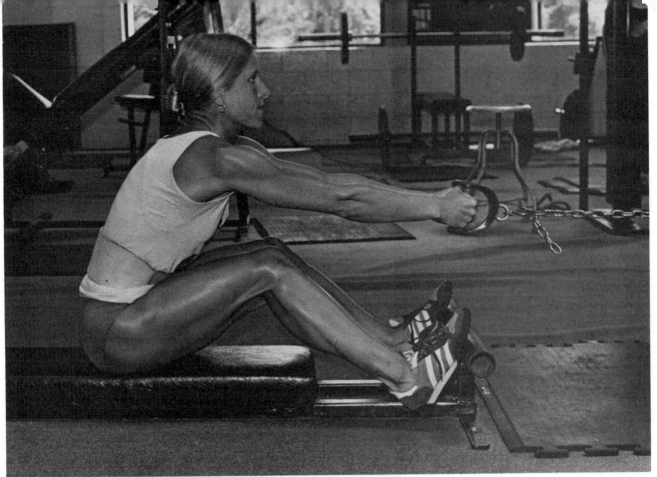

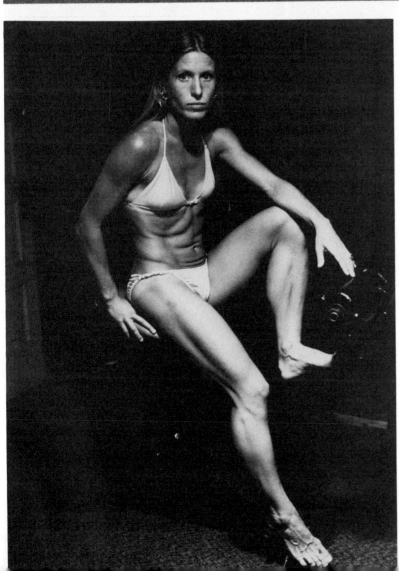

149

Q. How do you know if you've been training enough or overtraining? Sometimes I think I push myself too hard, but I'm never sure if I'm just wimping out, or if I'm really tired and should take it easy.

A. This is where a training diary is a must. When you wake up in the morning, be still in bed, and take your pulse for one full minute. Record this in your diary. This is your resting pulse. If you notice a rise in the number of beats per minute by more than eight to ten beats over what it was the day before, then that's a sign to get in an easier day.

Q. Is there a way to tell if the workout was hard other than just by the way you feel?

A. After I run, row, swim or cycle—and that's immediately upon stopping—I take my heart rate (put your fingertips directly over your heart to feel it, or under your jawbone halfway between your chin and your ear, counting for one full minute). This shows two things:

1. If the 10-second count for me is 32 beats, then I know that I have worked to my maximum heart rate. The American Heart Association says to find your rough maximum, take the number 220 and subtract your age. To figure out what this would be for ten seconds, I divide by 6.

   For instance, 220 minus 28 (my age) equals 192. To find out if my heart beats at that rate for those first 10 seconds, I'm counting after the workout, I divide by 6 (10 seconds being $\frac{1}{6}$ of a minute). That gives me $192 \div 6 = 32$. So a heart rate of 32 after my workout for the 10 count means I worked very hard.

2. Counting for the full minute tells more of a story. If my heart beat drops to under 100 beats for the whole minute, then it shows that my body was able to recover very quickly, and the workout was not that taxing. If my heart rate slows very little in that one minute after stopping the workout (say it's 160 beats for the full 60 seconds), then I know that not only did I work near my maximum heart rate (as the first 10 seconds told me) but my heart is not recovering quickly, so the next workout should be an easy one.

   If you'd like to learn more about this kind of thing, then I strongly suggest Kenneth Cooper's book, *Aerobics* (New York City: Bantam, 1970).

   P.S. And if you don't feel any pulse at all, get ready to sing the Hallelujah Chorus—you've made it to heaven!

Q. Should I eat or drink anything before exercising?

A. A few ounces of water (four to six) is a good idea to keep your body temperature down and keep your body in a hydrated state. Before a race, I'll drink an eight-ounce glass of water thirty minutes before and then take an additional mouthful of water about ten minutes before the gun goes off.

   I also have a tendency towards hypoglycemia (low blood sugar), and on rising in the morning I usually mix one tablespoon of nutritional yeast in a glass with diluted freshly squeezed lemon juice or grapefruit juice. I do this about one hour before I go out the door, and never feel it in my stomach during the workout.

As for eating before a workout—I absolutely never eat just before. Why? Blood flows into the stomach to digest the food. Now blood is vitally needed to bring energy and oxygen into the muscles. The heart then has to pump blood to the digestive organs as well as to the muscles, and this is a great strain on the heart. And if that's not enough, exercising right after a meal can really make you feel like you swallowed a stone. Hardly the set-up for maximum performance. I usually plan my exercise four to five hours after the last meal.

Q. Is it OK to drink water during a workout?

A. It used to be in style years ago for the coach to deny athletes water during a grueling workout to "make them tough." I've seen athletes faint from dehydration and heat exhaustion during these sessions, trying to become heroes in their coach's eyes—it's a dangerous practice.

Don't wait until you're thirsty to take a few sips of water. Your thirst mechanism can signal you when you've already downed one quart of water. Just be sure to sip the water *slowly.* Otherwise, you can be setting yourself up for stomach cramps, as well as the dubious delight of completing your workout with your belly feeling like an aquarium.

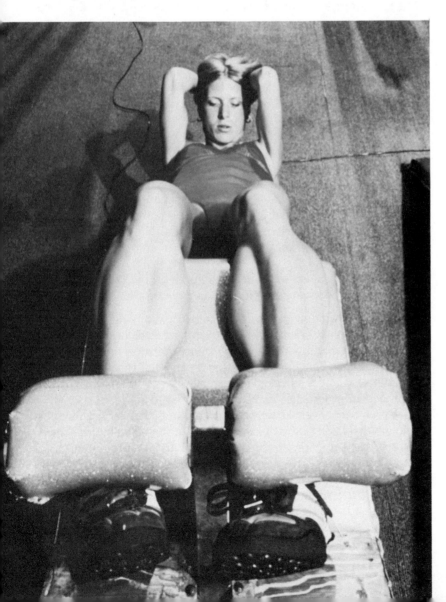

NUTRITION AND HEALTH

Q. What kind of diet are you on?

A. I've been a vegetarian for ten years now—mostly fruitarian. I'm a raw foodist. Since recent cytotoxic testing, my diet is even more strict, and I feel terrific. I am on a closely monitored (blood, urine and tissue tests regularly) vitamin and mineral program. In addition, I fast twice a month for two days total, and seasonally for four three-day stints. Other nutritional habits—never eat airline food, or eat late at night. Low-fat eating gives me the best athletic results. I don't drink alcohol. Favorites: garlic and ginseng—they really work for me.

Q. What do you do for a headache? Is there anything you can do except take two aspirin?

A. I rarely get headaches—in the last ten years I think I've had two. I'll share an ancient Oriental headache cure with you though—a remedy that I also use for pain of any kind. I've shown this to many women who have told me of menstrual cramps, and I've had quite a few letters from them telling me of their success with this. One woman tried it on her husband, who had a toothache in the middle of the night, and it worked. Needless to say, in cases of severe or prolonged pain, see your family healer.

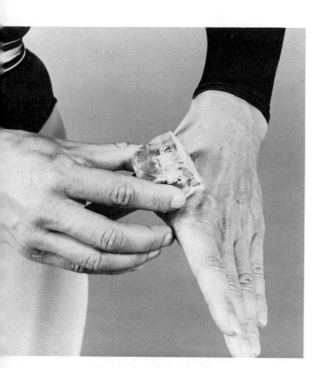

In the V formed by the index finger and the thumb, rub a cube of ice for ten minutes. The spot you want to pay attention to is approximately one inch in from the web of your hand.

This spot is a very powerful acupuncture point called the "Magic Window" by the Chinese, perhaps because stimulation of this point seems to cause pain to magically disappear as if through a window.

If you suffer from frequent headaches, you should ask yourself why, and try to alleviate the cause. Constipation, overeating, bad food combining and dehydration are a few commonly overlooked causes of headaches. Remember—the headache is only the symptom of something else.

Q. My daughter suffers from menstrual cramps and I'm reluctant to keep giving her pain killers for this. Is there another answer?

A. The "magic window" ice trick has helped a number of women who have menstrual cramps. As I said of the headaches though, the cramping is a symptom of a greater cause that must be discovered.

Has your daughter been tested for anemia? Have you had her mineral balances checked—especially the calcium/magnesium ratios. Her general health must be attended to first.

As a teenager, I was occasionally bothered by cramps but found that taking extra niacin and bone meal in tablet form helped me immensely. These I took for several days before the onset of my cycle, along with several tablespoons of molasses. A Swiss woman once quelled a formidable set of cramps for me years later with a brew of shepherd's purse and valerian root tea poured boiling hot over raspberry leaves and berries and served with honey. It was a very strong tea, but it worked quickly and I felt

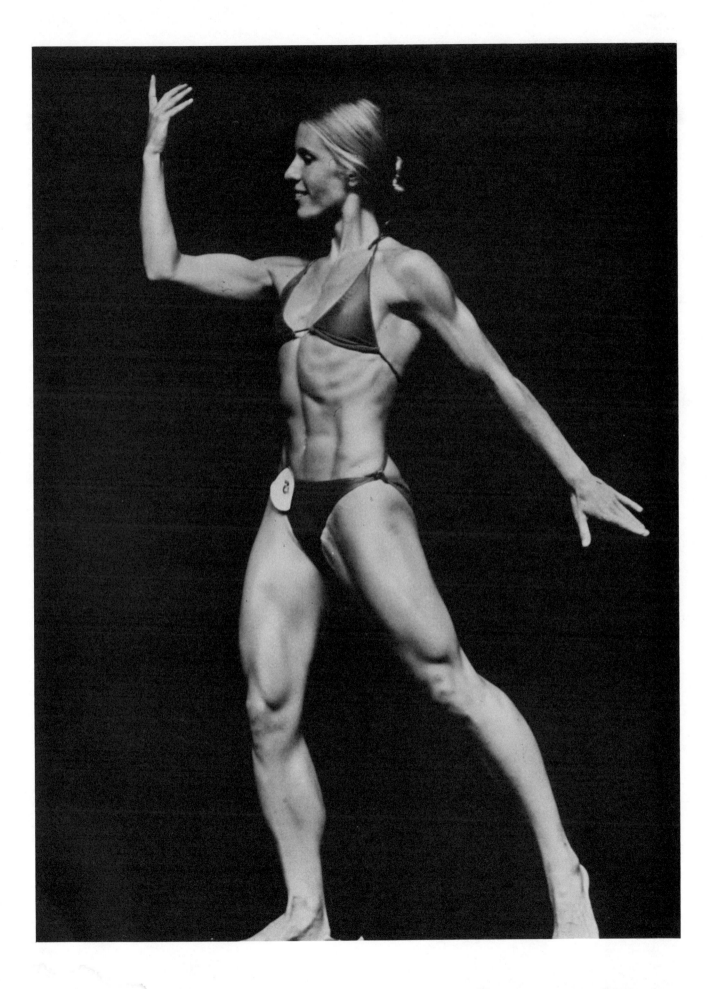

marvelous for the rest of the day. This was actually the incident that made me seriously take up the study of herbs and their healing effects. (See "Staying with It—Herbal Remedies" for more information.)

Q. My sneakers really stink! I hate to throw them out though. I paid $59.00 for them and they're hardly even worn out. Is there any way to get the smell out?

A. Your sneakers are suffering from a malady I call smell-o-vision! That is, you can smell 'em before you can see 'em. The answer: throw them in the washing machine with some strong detergent. You can't wear them the way they are, so if they shrink, it's a risk you're willing to take, right? And if you use a cold water setting, they probably won't shrink. Then, remove the insoles and throw them away. Dry the shoes in the sun, stuffing newspaper in them to help them keep their form. Put in new insoles and wear socks with your shoes from now on. Keeping your sneakers just for exercising allows them to dry out properly between sessions and prevents smell-o-vision. And if all this doesn't work, you can always hang them up and plant flowers in them.

Q. What can you do for muscle cramps?

A. Minerals to the rescue! Raw foods help to guard against mineral deficiencies, especially dark green leafy vegetables. Sea vegetables like dulse and kelp are another valuable mineral source. Vegetable juices of beet, carrot, celery and cucumber are not only refreshing but are mineral gold mines and a healthy alternative to cola drinks and other caffeine beverages that leach vitamins and minerals from the system. Alcoholic beverages can also set you up for muscle cramps by the same leaching effect and by dehydrating the body, so be warned—and reach for the carrot juice.

Q. Is coffee really that bad for you?

A. Yes, "caffeinism" is the new word that doctors are using to describe the nervousness, anxiety and insomnia caused by the caffeine consumption that can have psychiatric tie-ins. Caffeine is also found in other "food" substances such as chocolate bars, tea, soft drinks and many pain relievers and over the counter "wake up" pills.

Besides creating the nervous symptoms, caffeine causes other reactions which are focused on women. Painful breast lumps or cysts and breast cancer are now linked to caffeine. Women with histories of fibrocystic breast disease have had complete reversals in their condition when they stop using caffeine, as demonstrated in studies by Dr. John Minton, an Ohio State University surgeon. Birth defects, heart attacks, cancer and high blood pressure are all now linked to coffee. Caffeine is closely related to chemicals that involve DNA, our genetic material. And through DNA cell mutation and resulting cancerous tumors are formed.

Caffeine also leaches Vitamins E, the B complex and C as well as zinc and other key minerals such as calcium. The implications of this for an athlete in particular are obvious.

This is solemn news for chocolate, coffee and cola drink lovers, but there is some good news—abstention from these caffeine sources has produced reversal of the symptoms in clinical studies using humans. You may go through some initial withdrawal symtpoms, but then there is usually an increase in energy from having kicked the caffeine habit. In addition, there are now a variety of cereal-based coffee substitutes that might appeal to you. Finally, if you still miss that "pick-up" from the caffeine, try some of the herbal teas or ginseng tea. Your body will thank you.

Q. Does taking too much calcium give you calcium deposits?

A. No. A normally functioning parathyroid gland controls the necessary inverse ratio of calcium to phosphorous in the body. Calcium is used by the body as deposits when there is damaging wear and tear on a joint. The body would rather make the joint immobile by depositing calcium than have the joint wear out. Taking more calcium than necessary in supplement form would simply result in the excess being excreted.

Q. Is there any *one* vitamin I need the most, and if so, what is it?

A. Balance is what the laws of nature are all about. However, the experts I consulted on this all agreed on Vitamin C. This is the very least they feel a person should take.

Q. What happens if you take too many vitamins?

A. The water soluble vitamins—C and the B complex—are simply excreted. A, D, E and K, the oil soluble vitamins, if taken in huge quantities over an extended period of time, can be toxic. For further reading on this, I suggest *The Nutrition Almanac* (N.Y.: McGraw-Hill, 1975.)

Q. What is dessicated liver, and is it good for you?

A. Dessicated liver is free of external connective tissue and fat, dried in a vacuum at a temperature below the boiling point to conserve as much content as possible. Powdered or tablet form is usually one fourth by weight what the fresh raw liver would have been.

Is it good for you? It's high in copper, iron and other minerals as well as B_{12}. Keep in mind that the liver is the animal's chief detoxifying organ so that the steroids, antibiotics and other drugs used by the meat industry are *ingested* by this organ. I'm not a fan of liver for this reason, but if you feel you must eat it, do try to get non-American sources (Argentine beef is still free-ranging.) Liver is also not the complete hematinic or blood builder it's been cracked up to be all these years.

Q. What's your opinion on protein powders? Isn't this what athletes eat to get big and strong?

A. Please refer to the question on protein (page 156). I think protein powders used properly and not in excess can be an aid to some people. However, I disagree with the popular practice of mixing the powder with fruit juice. Fruit juice must pass out of the stomach quickly—most of the berry juices are actually digested in the large intestine rather than the stomach. In the presence of protein and fat, this quick passage cannot be accomplished, and putrefaction, gas and bloating occur. Not the ideal state to be in while preparing for a workout!

Q. Is it true that your stomach shrinks when you go on a diet?

A. No. The stomach secretes digestive fluids as necessary. When you eat less, it secretes less and feels smaller, but this is due to the smaller quantity of food it is digesting.

Q. How many meals do you eat every day?

A. I eat when I'm hungry, and when I'm not hungry I don't eat. I prefer four to six small snacks in a day over three large meals. This way, I feel that my metabolic fires will continue to burn all day and my system avoids hungry, low blood sugar blues.

Q. How do you figure out how much protein you've eaten in a day?

A. The Department of Agriculture publishes a marvelous book entitled *The Composition of Raw Food,* which is yours for under ten dollars from the Superintendent of Documents, U.S. Government Printing Office, Washington, D.C. 20402. This book lists hundreds of foods analyzed in detail according to protein, fats, and carbohydrates and other elements as well, including calories.

   Another excellent book is Frances Lappé's classic, *Diet for a Small Planet* (New York: Ballantine, 1971).

Q. Do herbs have side effects?

A. When we take herbs into our systems, we are dealing with two biological systems—ours and the plant's. Age, growing conditions, and time of harvest are a few factors that affect the herb's potency. Of course, our systems are changing second by second.

   Herbs can have side effects with some people sometimes. Too much of an antihistamine could cause dry nasal passages, for instance. Too much garlic or cayenne pepper could cause heartburn. Some side effects are obviously more annoying than others.

   Herbs must be taken with knowledge and moderation. They've been used for thousands of years by many cultures around the world as an aid to well being. Of course, there have been people who have abused certain herbs (opium for one) and paid the price. Herbs are nature's gift to us, to be used with prudence and understanding.

Some Precautions

The Little Herb Encyclopedia (Springville, Utah: Thornwood Books, 1980) offers these warnings about certain herbs for children and pregnant women.

Herbs During Pregnancy. Most herbs can be taken through the pregnancy with no ill effects. Many herbalists strongly recommend that some herbs *not* be taken during pregnancy. These herbs are black cohosh, pennyroyal, and any female corrective [hormone herbs] herb combination. Most of the hormone herbs are not used during pregnancy. But especially those mentioned above should *not* be taken.

Herbs for Children. Children can take most herbs with no adverse effects. Obviously, the dosages for medicinal herbs must be reduced since a child is much smaller than an adult. A general rule for determining dosage is to calculate the dosage according to the body weight of the child. Preschool children take approximately one fourth an adult dosage. From age five through ten, one half the adult dosage is sufficient. Early teens take three-fourths the adult dosage. When the growing child reaches adult size (sometime between the ages of thirteen and twenty), the full doses can be used.

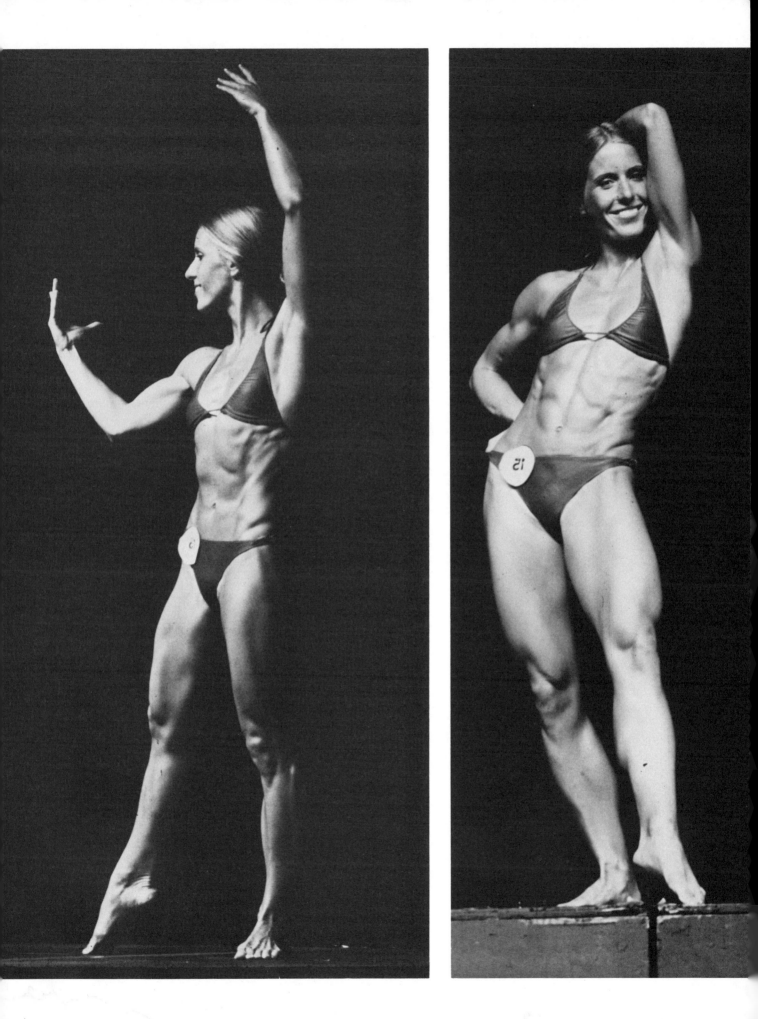

The only herbs to be cautious about giving to children are the hormone herbs. Ginseng, damiana and black cohosh should not be given to children before they reach puberty. Also, some of the strong laxative herbs and herb combinations should be used sparingly. Cascara sagrada is one herb that can have strong laxative effects for children.

Q. Do you think people should take vitamins?

A. Would you wake your dog up every morning and feed him coffee, a doughnut and a cigarette for breakfast? No. But many people think nothing of having a breakfast like that for themselves. Their dogs eat better than they do.

Nor would I put water in the gas tank of my car. It wouldn't run. You don't have to be fanatical, but I absolutely believe in vitamins. Our food is processed, picked green, sprayed with pesticides, fertilized with chemicals, stored in warehouses and packed in plastic. Something has to be lost from the food after all this. That's why I take vitamins.

Q. Do athletes need special nutritional supplements—more vitamins than other people?

A. Not really. In some instances increased Vitamin C or the stress vitamins (B complex). Running or cycling in polluted areas, I usually up my Vitamins A and C intake because they are antioxidant vitamins. For therapeutic reasons, I would also take specific other supplements. Remember, however, that vitamins should not replace meals. An insufficient diet supplemented by many vitamins does not let you off the hook in the eating department. North Americans are said to have "the most expensive urine in the world" due to excess vitamin intake, which is only excreted.

Q. What about supplementing minerals? Don't you have to replace all of the minerals you lose in sweat every workout?

A. Iron is an important mineral for athletes because it works in the transportation of oxygen. Potassium, sodium, magnesium and calcium are lost in perspiration. Here, the *balance* of these minerals is very important, and I have regular hair, urine and blood analysis to test the ratio of these minerals one to the other. Women tend to be iron deficient due to menstrual losses. Keep in mind also that great amounts of minerals are lost through cooking vegetables, and this is why I prefer eating my food raw—except of course for grains, which must be cooked to be digestible. Again, supplementing minerals does not replace good eating.

Q. Do you believe in carbo loading?

A. This diet was popularized by Ron Hill, the British marathoner of the late sixties, and it still has many devotees even today. I am not one of them, for several reasons, but let's discuss what carbo loading *is* before we discuss what it *isn't.*

Carbo loading is a five-day to one-week pre-race diet and exercise plan for endurance events such as the marathon.

A hard workout day is used to deplete the body's store of muscle glycogen. For the following two days, only protein is to be eaten, the idea being to starve the liver of glycogen and create an overabundant need for carbohydrate, which is met with nothing but all the pasta, bread and sweets you can eat for the next three days. Proponents of this plan claim that the body is then able to store 400 hundred percent more glycogen than usual, to be used on race day for greater performance.

Carbo loading in this fashion would be a disaster for anyone with hypoglycemia (low blood sugar). In addition, the protein phase of the plan can put the body into ketosis, which is a toxic state, and is also stressful on the metabolism. This wear and tear usually shows itself when the "carbo loadee" gets extremely irritable and negative, hardly a desirable state before a big race.

Also, the carbo-loading phase has been known to cause constipation and dehydration, because the carbohydrates need a tremendous amount of fluid for digestion and storage as glycogen, a need which is difficult to meet. Athletes tapering off their training during the final days prior to the big race often do not even feel the thirst because they're not sweating, and don't feel the need to drink. So they may actually go into the race dehydrated. Again not ideal by any point of view.

I feel that slightly increasing your natural fruit and grain intake two to three days before the race is fine. But don't expect quantum leaps in performance. The best strategy for any race is to do your training and be prepared.

Q. What is wrong with the modern North American diet today? Most people are getting three square meals a day, so what's the problem?

A. My observations have yielded six major faults of our typical daily fare:

1. There are too many refined carbohydrates. Because of this refining, there is far too little bulk. Bulk prevents constipation, which is far from being inconsequential—constipation can be the forerunner of serious problems down the road.

2. The North American diet is too high in protein and fat. Acid-forming foods are meat and cereals. Alkaline-forming foods are fruits and vegetables, which the primitive North Americans ate in abundance.

3. It lacks Vitamin C, which is one of the most essential vitamins. Linus Pauling, Nobel Laureate, has been outspoken on this topic.

4. The modern diet is too high in salt, too low in other minerals lost through overcooking and processing.

5. Our food is fragmented and therefore imbalanced. Early people ate the animal, including the internal organs—the *complete* chicken, including the bones; the *complete* fruit, including the skin. Now we process the food, take away all the nutrients, and then put only a few back and call it "enriched." White bread is a good example of this.

6. Our diet has too much saturated fat. Wild animals eaten by early North Americans had less saturated fat than our domestic animals—especially now with the meat industry's intensive farming methods. In the past the ratio of saturated to unsaturated fats was much better.

Q. Were our ancestors a lot healthier then because of this diet? Didn't they die young?

A. Let's face it, life was tough and short for our ancestors. Fossils even show that some of them had rickets. However, the diseases were different from those of today. Most of the epidemics were due to overcrowding and unsanitary conditions. Bubonic plague was carried by rats, for instance, and rat bites were quite common. There was also no refrigeration, so food handling was generally of an unhygienic nature.

Our diseases, however, are the diseases of civilization—diabetes, heart disease, ulcers, constipation, psychiatric problems and cancer. So while we don't have to worry about death by rat bite, the "good life" of ours is delivering us into the hands of what the ancients called the sword of Damocles—*coronary thrombosis.* I suppose there have always been a few flies in every ointment.

Q. What's the big deal with vitamins? Certainly there's always a variety of food available in this country—how can you miss?

A. Read these charts and see how easily essential vitamins and minerals can be depleted. The following is a list of some of the more common elements that can deplete the body of vitamins:

Element	*Vitamin*
Alcohol	B & C
Antibiotics	C
Aspirin	C
Barbiturates	B
Caffeine	B, C
Chlorine dioxide, a bread preservative	E
Light	B_2
Rancid fat	E
Smoking	C (25 mg per cigarette)
Stress	B, C, A

Some of the major minerals are depleted as follows:

Absence of fruit and vegetables; table salt; caffeine; boiling food; stress; diuretics	Potassium
Caffeine; oxalic acid	Iron
Alcohol; chemically fertilized food	Magnesium
Caffeine; imbalance of protein; table salt; refined carbohydrates; pasteurized milk; flouride	Calcium
Boiling food; refining of food	Trace minerals

Q. Not only are most of the athletes you see on TV self-proclaimed "junk food junkies," they even endorse the stuff. They seem to be thriving on their diets, so is it *so* bad that they eat terrible food? They're professional athletes, and it sure doesn't seem to be hurting their income!

A. Recent trends are that the tennis stars, for one, are barely out of braces when they bare their new orthodontic work on billboards and TV while holding the latest rage in junk food—be it fried chicken or some diet drink.

Moral considerations aside, they are young, and you cannot vindicate a diet by using young athletes as examples. If they were middle-aged or elderly and fat, then that would prove something.

Secondly, these junk food athletes perform well *in spite of* rather than because of their eating habits. They are supertalented.

There is no food in the world that's going to make you run faster, jump higher or throw harder. But good eating *can* help you to recover more quickly from the pounding of a fast run, the strain of jumping higher and the pain of throwing faster.

Arthur Ashe was a top-ranked tennis star at the time of his first heart attack. He survived it. He was in his early thirties.

Athletes of all abilities and talents often feel that their training gives them immunity to all the diet-related ills of our society. It doesn't work that way for most of us. Unfortunately, if you fly now, you have to pay for it later.

In the Olympics, you often see the "aged"—mid-to-late thirty-year-olds from Eastern Europe—beating our teenagers, especially in the endurance events. The lesson here may be that not being in the "paying later" phase of their careers as we see it here in North America, they can consummate their years of training with gold medals at the age when our athletes are retired.

Q. How can I really tell, as an athlete, if I'm getting enough vitamins and minerals?

A. Are you in poor health? Do you get sick before a big event, or after sustained hard training? Do you heal slowly from nicks and cuts and bruises? Is your skin not clear? Is your hair dry and full of split ends? Do you wake up more tired than when you went to sleep?

I use these questions, and any other little observations like recovery rate from hard training efforts and even dry skin, to tell me how my body's doing. I use blood, urine and tissue analysis to give me periodic information on my vitamin and mineral balances, and then adjust my eating and supplementation as indicated. Hit or miss tactics of "throw down some of this and maybe more of that" can be more miss than hit. As an athlete, you're a high-performance machine gearing for maximum performance, so why not get the "tune-ups," and be sure?

Q. Should the diet for an athlete be any different from that for regular people?

A. After years of self-experimentation, I've found that an eating plan high in complex *carbohydrates* (grains and raw fruit) improves my capacity for prolonged intensive exercise. I also tend to eat more *protein* than the average non-athletic person in order to help repair the muscle tissue that inevitably tears down under a heavy competitive workload.

Of the essential nutrients, this leaves fat and water. I've found a *low fat* diet (less than 15 percent of the total calorie intake) to work best for me. I've noticed that athletes with a high fat diet (usually junk food) have enormous difficulty performing in hot weather conditions. A high fat intake, especially with any kind of alcoholic intake (even if it's beer) causes a blood condition known as "hemagluttination." The red oxygen-carrying blood cells clump together, reducing their surface area, and thereafter reducing the athlete's oxygen uptake by a significant amount.

As a vegetarian, it's difficult for me to even consume high fat meals (unless I go crazy on peanuts). I usually advise athletes to at least cut down and eventually cut out their red meat consumption. The leanest steak can be 40 percent fat. I have them stick to broiled fish, white meat chicken and turkey without the skin. In this way, they get the protein without the fat. My prime protein source is tofu (see page 115 for example).

As for water, I drink it purified and lots of it. Living in the tropics I've consumed a gallon of water in a day, regularly. In cooler climates, you may not get that thirsty, but as an athlete, be sure first to replace water after a workout, before you start eating. Water helps to regulate your thyroid and keeps your body temperature stabilized, in addition, of course, to keeping you from being dehydrated.

Q. What's the quickest way to *gain* weight? My football coach says I need to put on at least fifteen to twenty pounds before I make the team this fall. How do I do it? I've got two months to get big.

A. Whether you're gaining or losing weight, the fastest way is the worst. There is no sensible way to gain weight that fast.

You want muscle, not fat, and unless you are still growing, forget it. It is unhealthy to ask you to gain that much that soon.

Unfortunately, your coach is equating size with strength. If you doubt that you can lose weight and get stronger, just ask Allan Paige and Lyle Alzado, two football superstars who dropped twenty pounds in the off-season and came back stronger and faster—to become All-Pro.

If you're up against guys who have larger physiques than you, make up for it in performance! Gaining twenty pounds of fat, you will sacrifice your speed and put a strain on your cardiovascular system, too. In the two months until your team try-outs, work on your speed (see speed exercises in the leg exercise section— Kangaroo Jump and Bounding—on pages 44 and 45), do a good strength program (emphasis on increasing poundage over the eight weeks). Taper off five to six days before the big try-out week, and then go for it! The working-out will have done an enormous amount more for you than if you had sat around eating, just trying to become enormous.

Q. How do you pick out a trustworthy book on what to eat? Some of them are so extreme: cases of eighty-five year old ladies doing the pole vault after eating some miracle health food.

A. 1. Look for mistakes in the book—if something you *know* about is wrong, then maybe things you *don't* know about in the book are wrong, too.
2. Are the percentages accurate? You'd be surprised at how often a list of the percentages add up to more than 100 percent!
3. Does the author contradict him/herself? You don't have to be an expert to spot this.
4. Is the book up to date? Some of those thin paperbacks in the health food stores are more than ten years old and on sale for half

the price most of the time because the information has since been proven wrong, and nobody ever bought them in the first place.
5. Is there some grasp of basic scientific logic by the author?

Q. Can you get too much protein? And is there any difference between getting it from animal or vegetable sources?

A. Any kind of excess protein, whether it's vegetable or animal, leaves a nitrogen fraction as part of the residue. Normally this is eliminated as urea by the body's kidneys. Of course, continual excess puts a strain on the kidneys, which may eventually damage them so they function less efficiently. Uric acid is also formed by some types of protein. The problem here is that uric acid that is not eliminated accumulates in the blood, and can lead to possible artery damage and rheumatic troubles. Urate deposits have been linked in some studies to hardening of the arteries.

So it's the old story of too much of a good thing becomes a bad thing. Protein helps calcium absorption, too much causes calcium excretion and osteoporosis can result.

Q. Then how much protein is generally recommended?

A. The rule of thumb used by most doctors and nutritionists is one gram of protein per kilogram of body weight (roughly one-half your body weight in pounds). So if you're 140 pounds, an estimated 70 grams would be a guide.

Q. Does *pure* mean good? You see it on all the labels now, and I wonder what it means—is it worth paying more for?

A. "Pure" is probably one of the most overworked words in the food industry—"pure" being used to describe unprocessed food that has no nasty chemicals added to it. The truth is, that the opposite may be the case. The natural food may contain a poison that is removed by processing. For example, raw cassava root contains cyanide. Processed cassava is edible as tapioca.

An "impure" food, however, is often superior because of the trace elements it contains. For instance, two of the purest things in most people's kitchen cupboards are white sugar and table salt —both considered to be avoided by nutritionists, doctors and food reformists alike.

So "natural" may not mean pure, and pure may not always mean good. The same goes for 100-percent natural granola bars, which can contain 30 percent sugar.

Q. My next-door neighbor eats every piece of junk food in the world but looks perfectly healthy to me—clear skin, and not overweight. Why?

A. In the Korean War and also in Viet Nam, autopsies on our soldiers revealed a high percentage of artery disease—these are eighteen- and nineteen-year-olds who had passed the medical exam and were physically fit.

Logically, we have to assume that the effects of a poor diet and lack of exercise would build up gradually over the years, so that many young people who appear to be healthy now could be on the road to trouble later.

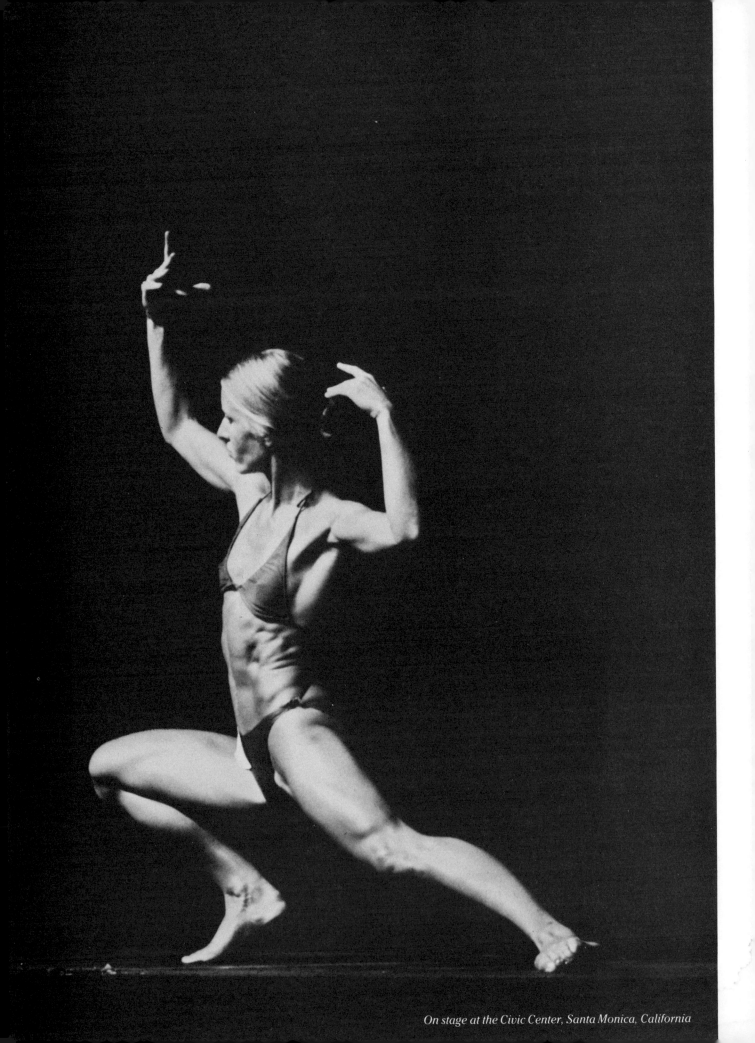

On stage at the Civic Center, Santa Monica, California

People who have problems early in life (e.g. skin blemishes, varicose veins, heart flutters) are in a sense the lucky ones because a problem is indicated, and they have been given warning so that it can be corrected.

But if you are rotting on the inside and OK on the outside, most people are lulled into a false sense of security, and it's only at forty or fifty years old, after the first heart attack, that their doctor says, "No salt, cut out fats in your diet. Get some exercise." Why not eat like that all of your life, exercise from the beginning and *prevent* that heart attack?

Q. What is the difference between fat and muscle?

A. You can't flex fat! Here's the technical breakdown.

	WATER	LIPIDS	PROTEIN
MUSCLE	70%	8%	22%
FAT	22%	72%	6%

Q. What is so terrible about frying food?

A. If you use an unsaturated fat, Vitamin E is lost, and prolonged frying may turn the fat rancid. Think of restaurants that use the same fat for weeks at a time in preparing french fries, for instance, and you get the picture. Also, when frying with saturated fat, burning of the fat contains acrolein, a poison.

Q. I'm confused—the magazine commercials claim that their products are polyunsaturated fat. What's the difference between that and saturated fat? Is there unsaturated fat too? And is one of them better for you than the others?

A. In a saturated fat, each carbon atom in the long chain molecule carries all of the hydrogen atoms possible. These fats are usually solid at room temperature, e.g. butter, lard, coconut oil.

Unsaturated fats are those in which one or more of the carbon atoms fail to carry all of the hydrogen atoms possible, and are usually liquid at room temperature, e.g., olive oil.

Polyunsaturated fats have more than one double bond in their molecular structure, and are found in fish, seed oils and other softer foods.

For the record, there are also mono-unsaturated fats—having only one double bond and common in both plant and animal fats.

Your body uses fats for energy and warmth. Most nutrition authorities agree that a healthy diet should include more unsaturated fats than the others. The reason? These fats contain factors called "essential fatty acids" that the body needs to synthesize Vitamins A, D and E. However, each type of fat is needed by the body in some degree.

EPILOGUE

The scene could be anywhere a journalist holds a microphone between us and asks the inevitable question: "To what do you attribute your win today?"

They want grand answers—wait for words like courage, bravery, determination, discipline. But the answer is simple and unglamorous. It doesn't conjure up visions of great battles lost and won, or do-or-die tactics. It's not even used in the hyperbole of television sportscasting, although it should be.

"To what do you attribute your win today?"

"To patience."

Plain old patience—the ability to wait, knowing that in the waiting, it'll be there for you—just as you imagined, only better, because you waited for it during all those long months of training.

When you plant a seed, do you dig it up every day to see if it's grown any yet? Nope. You leave it in that ground, water, pull the weeds and hope a little. You know you can't rush it—it'll grow.

Getting stronger is like that. You can't keep wondering if you're getting stronger. Plant that seed in your mind, do everything you can to go for it, and in the end you'll be there. You'll see. It'll even be better than you imagined, because you waited for it for a long time. You were patient, and you will also have discovered that strength is beautiful.

And that's what I wish for you—the beauty of your own strength, always.

Now, *Go for It!*

Gayle Olinekova

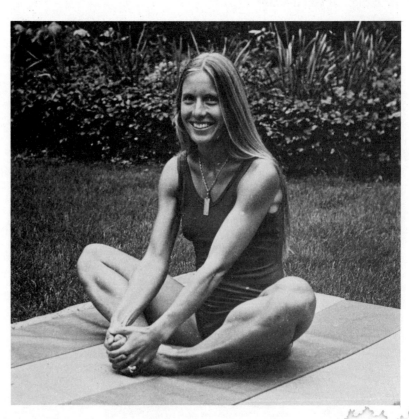